CW00326912

Fifty Shades

of Bondage & Submission

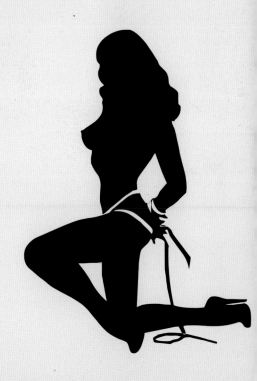

THIS IS A CARLTON BOOK

Published in 2012 by Carlton Books Limited
20 Mortimer Street
London W1T 3JW

10 9 8 7 6 5 4 3 2 1

A CIP catalogue record for this book is available
from the British Library.

ISBN 978 1 78097 298 5

Senior Executive Editor: Lisa Dyer
Managing Art Director: Lucy Coley
Copy editor: Nicky Gyopari
Design: Barbara Zuñiga
Production Manager: Maria Petalidou

Fifty Shades

of Bondage & Submission

A BEGINNER'S GUIDE TO BDSM

Renée Dubois

CARLTON
BOOKS

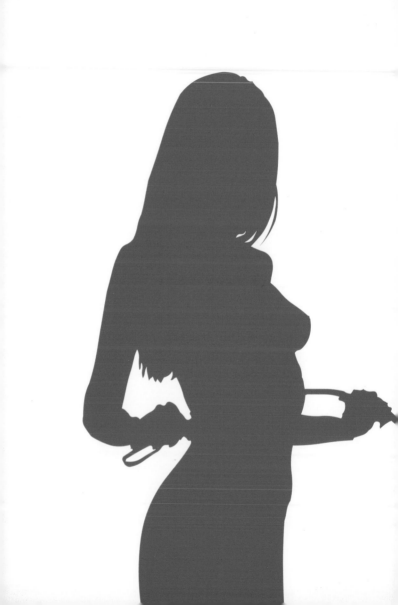

CONTENTS

INTRODUCTION

For so long deemed a deviant and controversial sexual practise, BDSM (an overall umbrella term that encompasses bondage, discipline, dominance, submission, sadism and masochism) has now entered the mainstream, in part thanks to the popularity of such books as *Fifty Shades of Grey* and *Bared to You*. If you are intrigued and interested in trying out some of the activities you may have heard about or read, but have no idea where to start, this beginner's guide will explain the basics of power play – how to establish rules and limits, how to roleplay and set a "scene" and how to engage in bondage, spanking and other games in a safe, sane and consensual (SSC) relationship with your lover.

Power play is not necessarily hardcore – it can be as subtle and sensual as pinning your lover down and caressing their body with a silk scarf – and it covers a huge range of activities, from light spanking or handcuffing to intricate rope bondage and heavy S&M practices. Engaging in BDSM play can help you open up to your partner about what really turns you on and express some of your darker impulses you may have kept firmly under wraps – which will only deepen your intimacy and desire for each other. So whether you simply want to break out of your everyday "vanilla" sex or have an inner goddess ready and waiting to crack her whip (or beg for mercy!), here's a wealth of ideas and advice to set you on a journey to a whole new world of wonder.

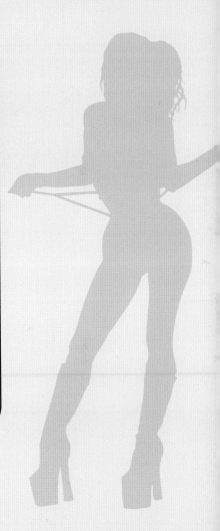

Safety Note: Some of the text in this book covers risky behaviour. This may not be interpreted as expert advice. In the event of an emergency or medical issue, always consult a doctor or healthcare professional. Whenever precautions and general first aid are mentioned and described in these articles, please be aware that every individual situation is different, that the information provided is of a general nature, and that all erotic power exchange play is always and only the responsibility of the partners involved.

POWER GAME
RULES

POWER GAMES ARE A PART AND PARCEL OF ANY RELATIONSHIP. THEY ONLY GET YOU IN HOT WATER WHEN YOU REGULARLY PLAY OUTSIDE OF THE BEDROOM. BUT A LITTLE CONTROL BETWEEN THE SHEETS? THAT'S A WHOLE DIFFERENT SHEBANG. AS LONG AS YOUR PARTNER IS GAME, THESE SCENARIOS CAN GIVE YOUR SEX LIFE A KICK.

BUT BEFORE YOU START MASTERING YOUR SLIPKNOT, YOU NEED TO SWOT UP ON THE RULES OF THE GAME. MOST PEOPLE THINK OF BDSM AS NO-HOLDS-BARRED, ANYTHING-GOES SEX PLAY. BUT GETTING TIED UP, WHIPPED, HANDCUFFED, OR EVEN MERCILESSLY TICKLED REQUIRES SOME BASIC GUIDELINES TO KEEP THINGS SAFE AND SEXY. EVERYTHING YOU NEED TO KNOW BEFORE GETTING DOWN TO BUSINESS IS ON THE FOLLOWING PAGES.

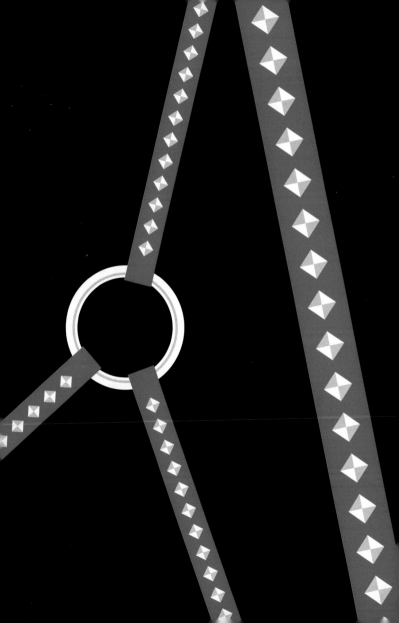

FROM ROLEPLAY TO BDSM

BDSM is a double-duty acronym that stands for bondage, discipline, dominance, submission, sadism and masochism – an umbrella term for certain kinds of erotic behavior between consenting adults. However there are many subcultures and the terminology can vary widely from your basic Sub (submissive, or bottom) and Dom (dominant, or top) to Femdom Mistress, Slave and even Lesser God!

For the beginner, power play is usually quite simple and starts with something like a bit of roleplay, spanking or using some new toys. Between existing partners, a BDSM relationship isn't necessarily fixed as they might dip in and out of the Sub/Dom roles as an exploration of their usual lovemaking. The power exchanges can also "switch" so that the Dom becomes the Sub and vice versa in one session or across several sessions. Although this kind of scenario is a light introduction to a much more involved relationships, it is one that's not going to frighten anyone too much! It also allows you to explore your fantasies and roleplaying in a safe environment with someone you trust. The main aspects to all power play are as follows:

Bondage: This usually involves some form of restraint combined with sensation play. The restraints can be anything from holding your partner's hands to very elaborate forms of rope-tying like Shibari. Sensation play can be as simple as a feather stroked across the body or as edgy as the flick of a whip.

Discipline: Discipline can be the chastisement, in whatever form, that accompanies bondage, but it can also be performed on its own, and is mostly concerned with control and obedience. It is frequently psychological, employing commands such as, "Kneel in front of me and don't move until I say so, Slave!" It usually involves punishment, such as spanking or paddling, for failure to comply with the commands or your contract (see also pages 16 and 24).

S&M: As everyone knows, sadists enjoy inflicting pain and masochists enjoy receiving, but the pain is meant to be "good" pain – the type that generates a glow throughout your body – and completely consensual.

Roleplay: Serious or light and playful, roleplay can enable you and your partner to experiment with different situations, whether teacher and pupil, doctor and nurse or police and criminal. For some, this helps act out deep-set emotions and fantasies in a safe setting.

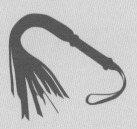

GETTING STARTED

Communication is the best way to begin with any kind of power game. Once you truly understand your partner's fantasies and desires, and they understand yours, lovemaking can become mindblowingly exciting and intimacy can deepen. Realize that human beings are complex and that power relationships can be explored in lovemaking while your day-to-day relationship is still one of mutually equal partners. It's about learning what you like, learning what your partner likes, and creating a situation, or "scene", that brings you both pleasure. Don't worry about how outlandish, silly or kinky your fantasies seem to be, or even whether you really want to do them. Sometimes even quite extreme fantasies can provide ideas to explore or help you understand what turns you on.

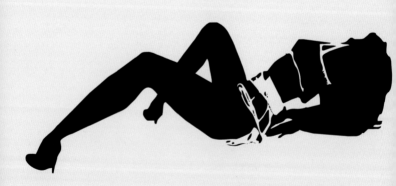

STARTERS' TIPS

- Get yourself in the right frame of mind. Consider this: If you're not ready to talk about your kinky thoughts, you're probably not ready to act on them.

- Start simple. Even if your ultimate fantasy is to create a home dungeon of bondage equipment, start by getting out a few scarves during your next romp and seeing your partner's reaction. If they seem freaked, they are probably more likely to come around if they think it's their idea. So claim that you were hoping to reenact the Dance of the Seven Veils – but now that they brought it up, it might be fun to try a little tie-up scenario.

- When you're ready to dive deeper, show rather than tell. There is a magazine for every desire under the sun. Try leaving one or two lying around (the bedside table is a good place) and thumb through it with your lover.

- Use the "friend of mine" gambit. This also works when you want to be subtle: "A friend of mine went out with this guy who liked to spank her and she said it was sexy." Along the same lines, use a study: "I read the other day that one out of every ten people has experimented with sadomasochism (true by the way), "that it is most popular among educated, middle- and upper-middle-class men and women" (also true), "that getting into kink shows that you're really comfortable with your sexuality and knowing what gets you off" (yup, also true), and that "it is like a cardio workout". OK, this last one is a bit of an exaggeration – you will burn more calories when you play rough because doing anything new jumpstarts your adrenalin, which in turn makes your heart pump harder. But how much you work it depends on your fitness level in the first place.

TOP OR BOTTOM?

Decide who is going to be the "top" (the one dishing it out) and who is going to be the "bottom" (the one on the receiving end). You may find you prefer doing the tormenting to being tormented. Or you may have a bit of both the pushover and the persecutor in you. Fine and dandy. In every relationship, the power dynamic is constantly shifting so why should it be any different in your kinky games?

To figure out which one best suits you, take out your pencils and get ready for a pop quiz. No cheating.

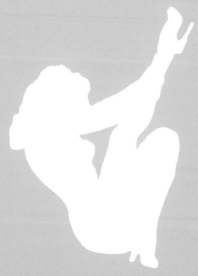

QUESTION 1

If you're in a restaurant with your lover, you:

A Sometimes order for them

B Don't throw a hissy fit if they order for you

C Don't mind who puts in the order as long as you get what you want

QUESTION 2

When you have sex, who usually makes the first move?

A Me

B My lover

C It's mostly 50:50

QUESTION 3

When you're in bed together, how do you normally lie?

A My partner cuddles me from behind

B I lie with my head on their chest or cuddle them from behind

C We lie close together with our arms around each other

QUESTION 4

How do you hold hands?

A My partner's hand is tucked into mine

B My hand is tucked into my partner's

C Our fingers are linked together

If you answered mostly As: You are so a "top"

If you answered mostly Bs: Stick to being a "bottom"

If you answered mostly Cs or a mix of As, Bs and Cs:
You're a switch hitter and can take as good as you get, so take turns with both roles (arm wrestle to decide, if you must).

COMMUNICATION &
CONTRACTS

Before you book a trip to the wild side of sex, you need to talk with your partner and make sure you are both on the same page. For example, is proper spanking ok or do you mean just a light tap? Is it ok if you pretend to be a meter maid whipping his sorry butt for parking illegally? Can he visit your back door?

You both need to agree on what kind of play you want to engage in. Yeah, it takes away some of the thrill of the moment but so does the shock of having your partner slap a muzzle on you and start commanding you to beg – if that isn't what you had in mind! Sometimes called a "Lifestyle" or "BDSM" contract, a terms of agreement can set out the duration of play (also called the "scene" or "session") as well as the type – you could set aside weekends only, for example, or have a full-on 24/7 relationship. Before you start drawing up a consensual contract, do some research online. The suggestions here are only ideas to get you started as no two contracts will be the same but every one should lay out the needs, wants, desires and benefits of all parties involved. Also realize that it is very unlikely that a BDSM contract will be upheld in a court of law, especially between a Dom and a Sub so the trust in all parties involved in the contract is critical. Here are some basic points to establish:

1. WHO IS IN CHARGE?

2. WHAT IS THE LOCATION AND DURATION OF YOUR "SCENES"?

3. WHAT WILL HAPPEN? DISCUSS THE CONTENT OF YOUR "SCENES".

4. ESTABLISH YOUR SOFT AND HARD LIMITS (SEE PAGE 20).

5. INCLUDE ESCAPE CLAUSES.
Due to the dynamics of this kind of sex play, there is always a chance the parties might outgrow one another, stop doing a particular activity or want to revert to vanilla sex only. An escape clause will let you reconsider.

6. SET A SAFE WORD AND HAND SIGNAL.
These are phrases for telling your lover to either slow down or stop altogether. Think of them as emergency brakes for when things get too tough, too scary, too painful, too annoying or simply too silly or boring. Plain old "Stop!" doesn't work as it can mean the opposite, so think of a word that you wouldn't normally use. Also include a hand signal, for times when you might be gagged! See also page 27.

BASIC TERMINOLOGY

Top: this is the person in charge – aka, Dom, Dominante, Master/Mistress.

Bottom: this is the person who gets to lie back and take it – aka, Sub, Submissive, Slave.

Switch: when you like to play both ways.

Vanilla: Someone who is not into BDSM, or sexual behaviour that does not encompass such activity.

24/7: when you're into a full-time erotic power exchange 24 hours a day, seven days a week.

TPE: total power exchange (think collar, leash and licking boots).

Squick: when you are turned off and about to reach your limit – the "ewww" factor.

SSC: safe, sane and consensual.

RACK: risk-aware consensual kink.

GGG: good, giving and game.

Scene: a time period of activities, also called play or a session.

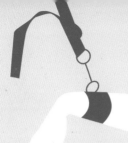

Subdrop: also called "subspace", this is the state of mind for a submissive who is so engrossed in a scene that they start to lose themselves. This is a state that needs to be closely monitored during every scene.

Aftercare: The time after a play session in which the participants calm down, discuss the previous events and their personal reactions, and slowly come back in touch with reality. BDSM often involves an endorphin high and very intense experience, and failure to engage in proper aftercare can lead to subdrop.

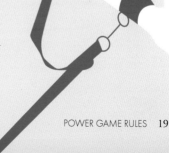

HARD AND SOFT LIMITS

There are two types of limits – hard limits and soft limits. A hard limit is something you will not do under any circumstance. It might include gagging, anal play or being turned upside down or spun when tied. Many limits are established by the submissive due to a value objection – either something that you feel is against your moral code or that you are squicked by (see terminology on page 18). Other limits are due to health objectives.

A soft limit is something that at this time you do not think you want to do, but perhaps your Dom can convince you. Or it may be something you will only do in a specific play situation.

How do you establish limits when you are new and don't know all the possibilities? You and your partner could tick off a checklist. There are many samples online, but see the list below to help you get started.

CHECKLIST

For each of the below questions assign a number based on this scale:

5 This is something I really like. Let's get it on!

4 Keen to try it.

3 I'm not sure, but it could be fun.

2 I'm not really into this, but if it excites my partner I'm up for it.

1 I don't think so.

0 NO WAY.

? I have no idea what you are talking about.

* Fantasy only, stays in my head.

☐ = on me, ◯ = on my partner

☐ ◯ Animal Roles
☐ ◯ Armbinders
☐ ◯ Blindfold
☐ ◯ Being Bitten
☐ ◯ Beating (soft)
☐ ◯ Beating (hard)
☐ ◯ Breast bondage
☐ ◯ Body bag
☐ ◯ Bondage (light)
☐ ◯ Bondage (intermediate)
☐ ◯ Bondage (prolonged)
☐ ◯ Bondage table
☐ ◯ Butt plugs
☐ ◯ Canes
☐ ◯ Chains
☐ ◯ Chastity belt
☐ ◯ Cock and ball bondage
☐ ◯ Cock ring
☐ ◯ Collars (worn in private)
☐ ◯ Collars (worn in public)
☐ ◯ Cuffs
☐ ◯ Dildos
☐ ◯ Double penetration
☐ ◯ Electricity
☐ ◯ Exercise (forced/required)
☐ ◯ Exhibitionism (friends/strangers)

- ☐ ◯ Eye contact restrictions
- ☐ ◯ Face slapping
- ☐ ◯ Fantasy rape
- ☐ ◯ Fisting
- ☐ ◯ Forced masturbation
- ☐ ◯ Gags
- ☐ ◯ Golden showers
- ☐ ◯ Hand jobs

- [ ] ◯ Harnesses (leather/rope)
- [ ] ◯ Hot wax
- [ ] ◯ Humiliation (private/public)
- [ ] ◯ Ice cubes
- [ ] ◯ Immobilization
- [ ] ◯ Intricate bondage (Shibari, etc)
- [ ] ◯ Kneeling
- [ ] ◯ Leather cuffs and belts
- [ ] ◯ Licking
- [ ] ◯ Masks
- [ ] ◯ Mouth bits
- [ ] ◯ Nipple clamps and clothespins
- [ ] ◯ Nipple weights
- [ ] ◯ Orgasm denial/control
- [ ] ◯ Paddles
- [ ] ◯ Riding crops/flogs
- [ ] ◯ Rituals
- [ ] ◯ Ropes
- [ ] ◯ Scratching
- [ ] ◯ Silk to be tied with
- [ ] ◯ Spreader bars
- [ ] ◯ Steel cuffs and chains
- [ ] ◯ Straight jackets
- [ ] ◯ Strap-on dildos
- [ ] ◯ Suspension
- [ ] ◯ Tickling
- [ ] ◯ Vibrators
- [ ] ◯ Video recording
- [ ] ◯ Voyeurism
- [ ] ◯ Whips

COMMANDS

o————————o

An important part of the Dom/Sub relationship,
commands and orders are executed by the Dom
to keep the Sub in line with the contracted play. Many
commands, such as "Stand up" have a hand command
that can be used in combination with the voice or alone –
just think dog training and you've got it! Here are a few
examples of the most common ones.

Stand (or Up): Stand with legs apart, and the arms at the side or
behind the back. Head up and eyes looking down.

Kneel: On your knees, with the back straight and arms behind the
back with the hand together. Head up and eyes looking down.

Kneel Spread: On your knees with the knees spread as far apart as
possible and feet meeting, breasts pushed out, and hands behind the
head. Head up and eyes looking down.

Sit: Sitting on the floor with crossed ankles, palms on knees and back
straight. Head up and eyes looking down. Or, as above but sitting on
a chair with feet flat on the floor.

Face Down (or Worship position): Knees tucked under chest with
head bowed and forehead resting on the floor. Hands straight in front,
by the head, palms down.

Lay Down Front/Back: Face down on stomach/Face up on back, with legs spread and arms above the head.

Inspection Stance: Stand with legs wide apart and breasts pushed out, hands locked behind the head. Head up, eyes looking down.

Punishment Stance: Standing, bent over at waist with hands grabbing ankles.

Go to Your Corner!: This is usually given for punishment, discipline or refocusing reasons. Kneel in the corner with the nose pressed to the wall.

Follow: To follow three or four paces back, to the right.

Heal: A leash command that can be used when unleashed. To follow one pace back to the right.

SAFETY ISSUES

The informed consent of all parties involved is essential in any kind of sexual play and even more so in any type of BDSM activity (see Contracts, page 16). Safe, Sane and Consensual (SSC) are the words most often used as the benchmark for agreement, which includes safe sex practises, not only that the behaviour involved is not a health risk but also that the risk of STIs is reduced. Pre-play negotiations should always include discussion of safety issues from both physical and psychological points of view.

Physical : Participants need to recognize that parts of the body could be damaged, that bruising, contusions and scarring can occur with the use of bondage practices and props such as crops and floggers.

Psychological : Intense sensory stimulation and fantasy power roleplay can have very strong emotional responses. Both parties need to be attuned to the needs and susceptibilities of their partner in order to be responsible for their health.

SAFE WORDS

Choose a safe word. This is a pre-agreed word or phrase that stops or slows down the amorous action when spoken by either partner. The basic concept is to allow either player to shout out things like "Stop, oh no, don't, you brute! Anything but that!" but knowing that they don't really want to stop the passionate proceedings.

Common safe words are "red" for stop and "yellow" for slow down, but the word can be anything you both agree on. Most people prefer something that wouldn't normally slip out (such as "No!", "Stop!", "I love you!", "Brangelina!"). Try not to make it something terribly long or hard to remember. "A tooter who tooted the flute, tried to tutor two tooters to toot" doesn't exactly trip off the tongue. Also, try to refrain from creating complicated systems. Using "green" for "great, get going with more of that" is fine; but using "blue" for "bring in the Berkley Horse" and "violet" for "tweezer clamps" is bound to confuse things.

If you're using a gag, make your "safe word" a "safe signal" – like a "thumbs up" or "thumbs down" gesture. Have the person hold something in their hand – if they drop it, it's time to stop. Or, if their hands or fingers are not tied up, these can be raised to put a halt to your hoopla.

BONDAGE SAFETY RULES

1 Choose a safe word and gesture (see previous page).

2 The one tie that you should never bind is one that causes any pressure at all around the neck. Nothing acts likes a cold shower on your love play like accidentally cutting off their air supply or breaking their windpipe. Also take care with gags if your lover is asthmatic, is prone to TMJ (Temporomandibular Disorder), has severe allergies, congestion, or any breathing problem (never stopping for breath when they talk is actually an argument for using a gag).

3 One is the loneliest number – especially in bondage. Though it is a hot fantasy to tie someone up in some precarious position (possibly with vibrators or other devices buzzing away) and then leave him or her to stew, in reality you must consider: What if the house is burgled? The room catches fire? There's an earthquake? Your mother arrives for an unexpected visit? They have to go to the toilet? The rule of thumb is to stay as close to your bound partner as you would to a baby left in your care so you can quickly release them.

4 Be prepared to cut your way out of any emergency with these two tools:

Safety shears: These are a must if you are using rope, fabric, or leather restraints. Don't use regular scissors – or even worse, a knife – for this. If you need to work quickly, the chances are you'll cut your lover with those sharp points and edges. Safety shears cost little and can cut through almost any material, including sheet metal.

Bolt Cutters: Handy for cutting jammed locks, padlocks and chains if necessary, as well as breaking into your local bank's vault.

What constitutes a bondage emergency? Start cutting any time your partner:

- loses consciousness
- has a freak-out panic attack
- experiences sudden, severe pain as a result of the bondage (this may mean a compressed nerve).

Don't hesitate - even if it's your most expensive locks or leather cuffs. You can always replace your equipment, but not necessarily your partner. Stay loose and easy - if you can't fit a finger between the restraint and the bound person's skin, it's too tight. Hands or other bound areas turning purple, getting pins and needles or feeling cold are also good cut-it-now indicators.

5 You don't have to be uncomfortable... unless you want to be. Certain bondage positions are more relaxing than others. Standing spread-eagled looks great but it can rapidly become tiring. Arms over the head are another sexy pose, but lead to shoulder strain when held too long. Some of the more comfortable positions include lying on a bed, tied seated in a chair or over the arm of a sofa.

6 Hold off on suspension poses until you have learned how, hands-on, from someone who really knows what they are doing. This sort of activity requires skill and practice.

- Avoid anything that puts any pressure AT ALL on the front of the neck. It can lead to unconsciousness quickly, as the carotid arteries go right to the brain.
- Never, ever, ever strike the head, neck, lower back (where the kidneys are), chest, backs of knees or abdomen. Continued internal (rather than superficial) pain several hours after a love session may indicate serious damage. Visit the doctor.

- Be careful with gags or very tight laces: Anything that restricts breathing can lead to suffocation – obviously not a good thing.
- If a position causes dizziness or nausea, stop and change direction – if you've been sitting, lie down; if you've been lying down, slowly sit up. This can also be a symptom of too-high temperatures, so lower the heat.

MARKS

You can't make an omelette without breaking eggs, and you can't take part in a heavy-duty pain scene and not expect to get black and blue. In order of bruising:

- Whipping, surprisingly, seldom causes marks.
- Spanking sometimes does.
- Caning always does, and bondage does more than you'd think.

You can avoid bondage bruises easily by covering the skin first before you put the ropes around and by taking care when releasing your partner (pulling rope over the skin may "burn" it). As for marks caused by hitting, try sticking to well-padded areas like the bottom, thighs and back if any substantial force is being used.

SIGNS

Cold, blue or white limbs are not an S&M fashion statement. They can be caused by a too-tight rope or a strap, by compressing certain veins or arteries with the weight of the body, or because the hands have been over the head for too long. It's not as scary as it looks (the average arm, leg, hand or foot can do without blood for 45 minutes) but it can be uncomfortable. Remove all restraints so the blood flow can resume (a little light massage never hurts at this point). And never leave clamps, rings or weights on for longer than 15 minutes.

WORST-CASE

A jammed bolt is the bad dream of anyone who takes part in a lock-up scene. The main thing is not to panic. Try a few more times. If you're still stuck, don't use a saw. Instead, soap up the skin – you may be able to slip out of your tight spot. Otherwise, you'll need a pair of wire cutters (available from most do-it-yourself or hardware stores).

Bad Dream Number Two is the possibility of losing something up the bum. Most things will make their own way out given the chance (you could try taking a laxative to ease things along). Avoid this in the future by never inserting anything all the way. And while you're at it, never insert anything that is sharp-edged or breakable and always use plenty of juice. If there's more than a spot of blood and/or pain after anal play, you'll need to get medically checked out.

WAX XXX

The burns from wax drips can feel sizzling sexy – or they can make you scream "Ye-ouch!" To stop wax from getting too hot, always use plain paraffin candles or ones specifically made for dripping on the body (rather than the kind made for creating atmosphere in a room). If the temperature of your play gets too blistering, cool the burned area with cold water (not ice – it will add to the burn) for one minute or more; don't apply petroleum products or any greasy lotions or butter.

◊
◊ **Warning: None of the above should be considered**
◊ **medical advice.**

THE MISTRESS
& MASTER MANUAL

You get to order him around and have an orgasm…
Or reverse the role!

Greet him dressed in black leather from head-to-toe,
stilettos and holding a small paddle or whip. Tell him
he has three minutes to get undressed or risk getting
punished. Punish him anyway. You choose – you can
make him your plaything or order him to ravish you from
head to toe.

Practise orgasm control – his. Stroke him but forbid
him to climax. Enjoy taking your time with your willing
victim – drive him to distraction and bring him to the edge
of ecstasy, then back off and make him plead for more!

Up the dominatrix ante – first tell him to do the
laundry, cleaning and all of the other household chores.
Then, stroke him and forbid him to climax. Want to
really make him squirm? Then tie him up and go to town
pleasuring yourself. He can't touch until you release him.

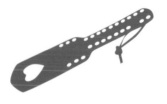

NO EQUIPMENT NEEDED

You don't have to own a wardrobe of latex or master more than the basics of the lingo to get into the pain game.

- A simple "Don't move an inch" may be the only restraint you need. Mix in some gentle scratching, pinching and a few light bites and you're playing with power.

- Get things started by lying spread out and telling your lover to do what they will. Then spell out the following scenario: he turns you around, holds your wrists behind your back with one hand, and wraps his other hand around your hair, lightly pulling it while penetrating you, doggy style. After a few minutes, he withdraws, turns you around, places a hand over your neck and goes back in for more.

- Take turns tying each other up spread-eagled and buzzing various pleasure points with a vibrator. Stop and make them beg for more.

- Order him to take off your high-heeled boots and caress your feet. Then tell him to take his hands higher.

- Pros use foot-suspension stirrups to get a hot head-rush, but standing on your head works the same magic. Spread your legs for a little oral action at the same time and the real torture will be seeing how long you can last.

Sub/Dom Names: One idea to help keep fantasy separate from reality is to give each other new names that reflect your power roles. Miss Birch might be great for a female dominant whereas Mr Grey is a popular male dominant choice!

TO LOVE AND OBEY

Sometimes all you want is unadulterated raw sex… with someone else in charge. Here's how to submit instantly – no experience necessary.

- Greet your love master with a deep curtsey that exposes your heaving, corseted breasts, giving him a teaser of what's to come. Guaranteed, he's going to respond with eager-beaver enthusiasm. Or back yourself into a corner and be ready to bolt when your lover closes the door. If he wants you, he'll have to chase you down.

- Find an outfit that makes you feel the role – a particular pair of boots, a certain lipstick colour, a bustier, a French maid's outfit. Get dressed up and ready to play.

- Tell your love tyrant that you've been very, very bad and deserve to be punished. Or try honing his bad-boy persona by encouraging him to sound off and use dirty talk. Tell him you want to be his dirty little girl.

- Encourage him to act as though he's in charge. You need to know that the very sight of you makes him so lust-driven that he can't contain himself. And as his love-thing, you can't refuse. So if he wants to come up behind you while you're washing up and pull down your knickers, there's nothing you can do but lay back and take it.

Warning: Never use dominance games to work out a problem in your relationship or to take out your anger on a submissive. If you have a conflict, resolve it by talking and don't let it get mixed up in your roleplaying.

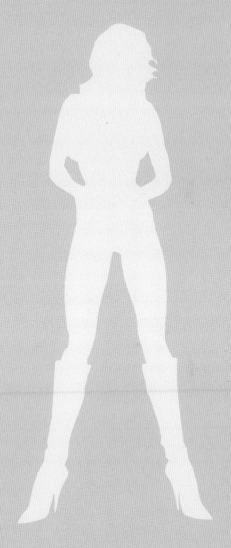

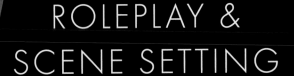

ROLEPLAY &
SCENE SETTING

ROLEPLAYING (PRETENDING YOU ARE SOMEBODY ELSE) GIVES YOU A CHANCE TO INDULGE IN SOME IMAGINARY GAMES AND PLAY AT SOMETHING DIFFERENT FROM YOUR USUAL BEDROOM PERSONALITY. IT IS ALSO A GREAT INTRODUCTION TO MORE EDGY BDSM SCENE-SETTING. ROLEPLAYING CAN, IN FACT, ACTUALLY TIGHTEN YOUR LOVE BONDS. WHILE TRYING ON A PERSONA DIFFERENT FROM YOUR USUAL DAY-TO-DAY SELF IS MOSTLY ABOUT GIVING A RACY REFRESHMENT TO YOUR USUAL ROMPS, IT WILL ALSO HELP TO BUILD TRUST BETWEEN YOU AND YOUR PARTNER, AND DEEPEN AND ENRICH YOUR RELATIONSHIP. AFTER ALL, WHAT COULD BE MORE REVEALING THAN ACTING OUT YOUR FAVOURITE SHIVER-ME-TIMBERS CAPTAIN HOOK DAYDREAM?

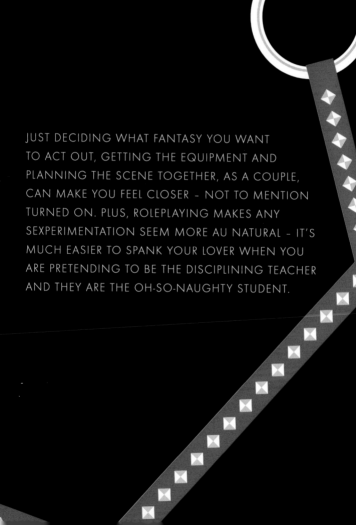

JUST DECIDING WHAT FANTASY YOU WANT
TO ACT OUT, GETTING THE EQUIPMENT AND
PLANNING THE SCENE TOGETHER, AS A COUPLE,
CAN MAKE YOU FEEL CLOSER – NOT TO MENTION
TURNED ON. PLUS, ROLEPLAYING MAKES ANY
SEXPERIMENTATION SEEM MORE AU NATURAL – IT'S
MUCH EASIER TO SPANK YOUR LOVER WHEN YOU
ARE PRETENDING TO BE THE DISCIPLINING TEACHER
AND THEY ARE THE OH-SO-NAUGHTY STUDENT.

PREPARATION

○━━━━━━━━━━━━━━━━━━━━━━━━━━○

Most roleplay fantasies can be played out without ever leaving your house – or even your bedroom, for that matter. After all, it's where your mind takes you that gives this sort of game-playing its spice. But the more props, decorations and other items you add to give your scene a realistic edge, the easier it will be to stay in role. So if you are in a harem, load the room with cushions. If it's more of a hotel atmosphere you are after, remove all personal items from the room. For a dungeon, display the floggers, whips and bindings you intend to use. But be realistic – if you have a pirate fantasy in mind, a toy scabbard slipped between the legs to part them could be highly erotic. A real scabbard, on the other hand, might result in a visit to Emergency.

Consider music, fragrances and lighting too – for example, incense, candles and background chanting are ideal for a Goddess setting, whereas some goth music and candelabras with dripping wax could be great dungeon scene-setters.

Ensure you have everything you need to hand well before you begin. There's nothing so mood-busting as having to scramble around to find lube, vibrators, cuffs and nipple clamps (see also Devious Devices, pages 50–65)! If you need specialist equipment for a certain scene, make sure you've bought and/or assembled it.

TIPS

- Set aside a designated time and place for your activities.

- Negotiate what you're willing to do ahead of time. Start by limited use of props, gradually adding more in subsequent sessions as you become more familiar with each other and the situation.

- Prepare for emergencies. Have a first aid kit, fire extinguisher and a torch (flashlight) nearby.

- Avoid toys that have sharp edges or corners – props should be carefully rounded off.

- Use plain paraffin wax candles not beeswax; beeswax have a high melting point and can cause burns.

DRESSING UP

Props and costumes will make it a whole lot easier to shimmy into your chosen character. Besides, it's lots more fun to get into fancy dress than to wear your everyday clothes when roleplaying. After all, this kind of pretend sex should never be a quickie.

From your undies to your coat (and especially the shoes), dress appropriate to your role. Once you have decided who you want to be, raid your closet. Chances are, you already have lots of outfits that can double up. But if you do need to add some bits and pieces, hit up the charity shops for items like miniskirts, blouses and shirts. Discount stores are the best place to grab inexpensive, body-hugging clothes (maybe even choose a size smaller than you normally wear), lingerie, thigh-high stockings and fishnet hosiery.

If you want to go all-out or need a specific uniform, shop post-Halloween for the best bargains. Dominatrix and fetishwear is very easy to find and sex-supply shops like Anne Summers (www.annsummers.com), Love Honey (www.lovehoney.co.uk), Temptations (www.temptationsdirect.co.uk) and Tabooboo (www.tabooboo.com) all have a huge selection of costumes in pretty much every theme imaginable. Toy stores are another good source for costumes as well as inexpensive props like handcuffs, hats, badges, fake guns and swords and other titillating trimmings.

Also, accessorize, accessorize, accessorize. Wigs, gloves, jewellery, ties, hats, glasses, wings, boots and bags not only put those oh-so-seductive finishing touches to your look -- they can be used as instruments of seduction. Think of what you can do with a pair of stockings or a leather belt. Mmmm.

Keep things just this side of real by making sure that you stock up on the tools of your trade. Business people need briefcases, teachers need rulers, cops need handcuffs, doctors need stethoscopes, pilots need hats, cowboys need lassos, porn stars need big boobs (this is where that push up bra comes in handy!)...the list goes on. It's up to you how close to reality you want to get.

SCENES

Just like the theatre, creating a good scenario requires drama, suspense and an element of surprise. You need to provide a plot and script, a set, props, costumes and effective acting. Here are some basic steps to get you started. Many BDSM scenes are organized along this very simple plotline:

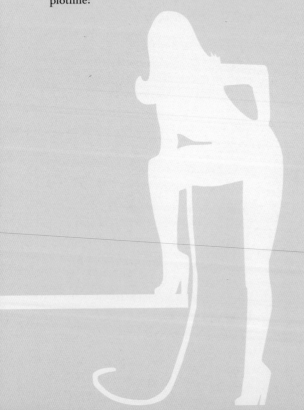

THE DOM ESTABLISHES AUTHORITY

The Sub, or bottom, needs to know that the Dom, or top, has unquestionable authority over him/her. This stage is when the actual fantasy situation is set up, whether it's his experienced Christian Grey to her virginal Anastasia or her Queen to his Slave. Maybe you're the queen who needs to test the slave in feats of endurance in order to decide whether he is worth keeping? Or maybe he's the police officer who's apprehended you shoplifting.

THE SUB TRANSGRESSES

At this stage, an explanation of the exact "crimes" is given to the Sub and they are informed of the penalty for each one.

PUNISHMENT

This can take any form, from verbal chastisement and posture stances to spanking and bondage, but the Dom should know what embarrasses or humiliates the Sub most and play on it.

SATISFACTION

For some Subs, the punishment is the release, whereas others might want to provide some pleasure for the dominant, or have the Dom comfort and pleasure them. Orgasm is almost always the end aim of the session.

BEGINNER'S STEPS

1 The Dom starts by telling the Sub to do exactly as they say, and that absolutely no deviation from those commands is permitted. The Dom then undresses the Sub and has them lie down with arms overhead and eyes closed. They are not to move, squirm, or open their eyes no matter what. The Dom then explains, in detail, precisely what they intend to do, and how much pleasure it will give them to take possession of the Sub's helpless body.

2 The Dom can then work in some sensory teases, running their fingernails lightly up and down their victim's body, paying close attention to sensitive areas that normally don't get touched very much, such as the undersides of the arms, thighs, face and neck. They should take their time, and be on the watch for any movement from the Sub – the idea is that they are being restrained by sheer force of will. So if they move, the Dom should sternly tell them that they're breaking the rules, followed by a quick nipple twist or slap to the inner thigh for emphasis.

3 Once you're both up to speed with the dirty talk and sexual commands, ramp up the action with a little actual bondage. Restraining the hands is the best way to begin – it immediately restricts freedom without making the person being tied feel totally helpless. But if you prefer to begin at the bottom with the ankles, go for it.

The important thing is to keep it just between the two of you. Don't include ties to the bed or a chair or a suspension bar just yet. The person being bound needs to feel confined, not cemented in place. They want to know that they can escape if they need to (at first, anyway).

4 Once you're comfortable with how things are, you can move on to more simple ties on pages 72–81. After that, you've earned your bondage badge and can take your pick of ties, restraints and positions.

INTERMEDIATE STAGE

So, now what? What does one actually do with a partner who's at your mercy, bound to the bed?

1 Before you do anything, slip a blindfold on them. Covering the eyes increases the sense of powerlessness and anticipation still more.

2 Then sit. Drive them out of their mind not knowing what's to come – or indeed, whether you're even still on the premises.

3 After a few minutes, quietly slide over and begin with a thorough body massage, with just a hint of kink. Pour some massage oil along your partner's body, or better still, use some body wax candles, which burn cooler than regular candles and turn into massage oil when you pour the hot drippings on to your partner's body. Straddle your partner and give them a very long, sensual massage. Work your way down their body, paying special attention to love buds. Keep going south, lingering over their inner thighs, teasing but not quite touching their hot spots.

4 Now make things a bit more interesting. Slide an ice cube over various places – sides, feet, arms, chest, belly, thighs, hands, in rapid and unpredictable succession, leaving it in contact for longer and longer periods of time. Keep reinforcing the "don't move" order.

5 Talk to them as you play. Tease them with little suggestive comments, or investigate how they're enjoying things. Take requests, if you do such things. Most of all, be sure they know you're having a down and delightfully dirty time. But don't talk incessantly; shut up occasionally and do your job.

6 Just when they're getting numb to your cool touch – and the ice cube has melted to a chip – switch to something with a sharper, more pointed sensation. You can use a bamboo skewer, toothpick, comb or, if you're a gadget person, a Wartenberg wheel – a wheel of prickly little pins that can be rolled over a person's skin. The contrast between the ice (which your partner is expecting) and a very different kind of sensation (which your partner isn't) should make them moan (and jump, giving you a chance to indulge in your Master and Commander role and warn them, with a slap to the sensitive inner thigh, that you did not give them permission to move).

7 Keep mixing up the stimulation in unpredictable ways. Your MVP (Most Valuable Player) here is the senses – all five. Even the most minor of sensory plays – like a quick kiss on the belly – can feel excruciatingly good when it is unexpected. See the Sensation Play chapter on page 114 for more ideas.

CLASSIC SCENES

Here are eight scenes to get the action started. All of these roles are unisex so you can switch parts. One word of caution: avoid characters and scenarios that are complicated, or that you're not familiar or comfortable with, or you'll spend more time on the prep than the play.

Stripper/Customer: The stripper can touch the client, but the client can't touch the stripper – except to tip.

Hooker/Client: Go high-class or down-and-dirty. Either way, the hooker does all the work.

Porn Star/Director: Pretend to be working with your favourite star, giving them very precise directions on how to please themselves.

Older Lover/Inexperienced Partner: Play an older, experienced lover dominating a shy young playmate, teaching them how to have fun between the sheets.

Employee/Boss: Be the stern boss and teach your employee a lesson in – er – leadership.

Patient/Doctor: Play the medic who gets seduced by their randy patient. Another take is to be a sex therapist unsuccessfully trying to cure a sex fiend.

Teacher/Student: Your wayward pupil has been naughty and needs to be punished.

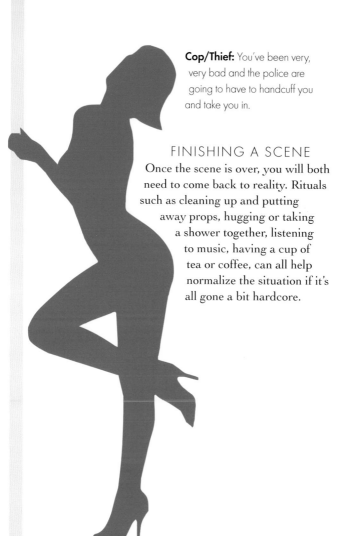

Cop/Thief: You've been very, very bad and the police are going to have to handcuff you and take you in.

FINISHING A SCENE

Once the scene is over, you will both need to come back to reality. Rituals such as cleaning up and putting away props, hugging or taking a shower together, listening to music, having a cup of tea or coffee, can all help normalize the situation if it's all gone a bit hardcore.

DEVIOUS DEVICES

SEX TOYS CAN ADD A WHOLE NEW DIMENSION TO YOUR LOVEMAKING. ALTHOUGH THERE'S A LOT MORE TO PROPS, TOYS AND TOOLS THAN YOUR AVERAGE VIBRATOR, MANY OF WHICH ARE DESCRIBED IN THIS CHAPTER, DON'T DISREGARD THE TRADITIONAL JOY BUZZER! AVAILABLE AS SMALL POWERFUL BULLETS THAT CAN BE LOADED INTO COCK RINGS, PLUGS OR STRAP-ONS, OR THE BIGGER RABBIT VIBRATORS, THEY HAVE LOTS OF USES, WORK ON BOTH MEN AND WOMEN AND CAN HELP ACHIEVE A MORE INTENSE CLIMAX.

SOMETIMES THE BEST SEX TOYS ARE THE IMAGINATION. ROLEPLAY USING COSTUMES AND GAMES CAN TURN SECRET FANTASIES INTO REALITY.

A LITTLE BONDAGE AND S&M
PLAY CAN BE HAD WITH SIMPLY
THE ADDITION OF BLINDFOLDS,
HANDCUFFS AND A LITTLE A WELL-
EMPLOYED PADDLE, OR TRY OUT
SOME OF THE MANY OPTIONS
DESCRIBED ON THE FOLLOWING
PAGES, FROM ROPES, GAGS AND
CUFFS TO CLAMPS AND HARNESSES
TO WHIPS, TICKLERS AND FLOGGERS.
IF YOU FIND YOUR INTEREST GROWS,
DECK OUT A SPARE ROOM AS A
PLAYROOM WITH BONDAGE AND
SUSPENSION FURNITURE, SUCH AS A
SWING, BENCH OR INVERSION TABLE!

Anal Beads: You stick these jewels in your bum and then pull them out again, one at a time. The beads get increasingly larger in size along the length.

Armbinder (aka single or mono glove): A restraint device consisting of a long sleeve into which both arms are placed, often fitted with laces or straps to hold the arms securely together.

Ball Gag: A gag – consisting of a ball, usually made of rubber, which is attached to a strap. The ball is placed in the mouth and the strap is placed around the head to hold it securely in place.

Ben Wa Balls: Small weighted balls, traditionally made of solid metal but also available in silicone, plastic or rubber. They may or may not have a retrieval cord on one end. They are inserted into the vagina to enhance stimulation. Duotone balls contain a smaller weighted ball inside that rolls around during movement to cause vibrations.

Berkley Horse: A type of suspension bondage furniture consisting of a padded bench with restraints and a pair of "arms" to which a person's legs can be affixed.

Blindfold: Plain leather, silk, padded or PVC, there are endless options… of course a plain silk scarf or men's tie would just as easily do the trick!

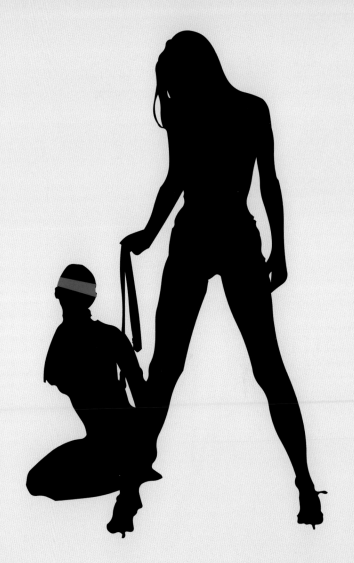

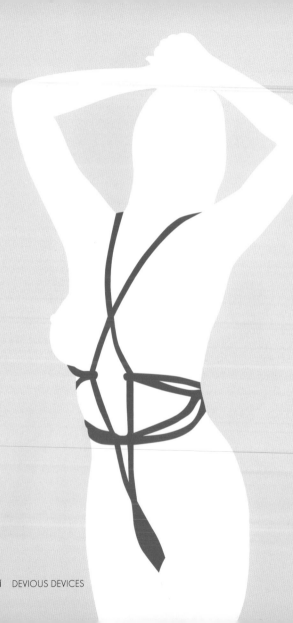

Body Bag: A long, heavy bag, often shaped like a narrow sleeping bag and typically made of canvas, rubber or latex, used to restrain a person very tightly. Sometimes includes integrated straps that wrap around the person within the bag.

Body Harness: A harness consisting of a series of straps designed to be worn around the torso, which may optionally include a mechanism for locking the harness into place and may also include rings or other attachments for ropes, cuffs or chastity belts. Neigh!

Bondage Belt: A belt used to restrain a person, which consists of a heavy band of leather or a similar material that can be strapped or locked about the waist and which has several attachment points to which the subject's wrists may be bound. For those who are all thumbs.

Bondage Mitt/ Mitten: A fingerless mitten, often made of leather, canvas, heavy vinyl, PVC or similar materials, which is placed over the hand and then fastened in place with an integrated buckling or locking cuff. The bondage mitt holds the hand flat or balled up, and prevents the wearer from being able to pick things up or otherwise make use of his or her hands. So don't expect any frisky finger moves.

Bondage Tape: A vinyl tape material, available in many colours, which sticks only to itself but not to other materials such as skin or clothing, making it ideal for bondage – and Christmas gift-wrapping. Use it to bond, blindfold, gag and restrain. It's easy to remove and unlike regular tape, won't hurt.

Breast Press (Breast Clamp): A type of device, often consisting of two horizontal wooden planks with an adjustable screw or clamp mechanism between them, which can be clamped over the breasts – turning her into a mammary sandwich.

Bullwhip: A type of single tail consisting of a woven or braided leather whip, usually longer than 1.2 m (4 ft) and sometimes 1.8 m (6 ft) long or more, with a short rigid handle. You'll need to be a real cowhand to handle this baby properly. Yeehaw.

Butt Plug: A sex toy designed for anal penetration that has a flared base. Usually smaller than a typical dildo and not shaped like a penis, it is used to give the wearer a very "full" feeling. For those seriously into roleplaying, there are versions with fox, bunny and pony tails for "animal roleplay".

Butterfly Chair: A chair that contains two horizontal planks to which the legs can be secured. It is affixed to a pivot so that the legs of the secured person can be spread apart. Otherwise known as a visit to the gynaecologist.

Cable Loop/Slapper: A tool used for striking, consisting of a loop or occasionally two loops of thick wire, coated with plastic, rubber or leather, and affixed to a handle. A cable loop can be used much like a crop or similar implement, and produces intense sensations and really good reception.

Cable Tie/Cuff: A type of cuff consisting of a thin plastic strip with a row of teeth in its surface, and a small ratchet on one end. The end of the cable tie can be placed through the ratchet to form a loop, which can be pulled tight but not loosened again. Sometimes used by police instead of handcuffs. Remember to have scissors handy.

Cat: Not your household pet or the new orgasmic version of missionary. Instead, this is slang for a cat-o'-nine tails, a specific type of flogger consisting of a handle, often made of wood and wrapped with cloth, with nine lashes affixed to it. The lashes, usually made of rope or of leather, are braided or knotted.

Chastity Belt: Any device intended to prohibit contact with or stimulation of the genitals. Female chastity belts often take the form of a lockable harness that passes between the legs and around the waist; male chastity belts may include a locking enclosure into which the penis is placed. You know he isn't a cheating liar when he slips into one of these.

Cock Ring: A ring (often made of metal or rubber) or strap that's designed to be affixed around the base of an erect penis. The ring allows blood to flow into the penis but constricts the penis sufficiently to prevent blood from flowing out, preventing the penis from becoming flaccid once it is erect. Now she can lead him around.

Collar: An item worn around the neck, sometimes equipped with a locking device to prevent its removal, and often worn as a symbol of submission. Special "posture" versions keep the neck upright, helping to create an attentive stance. A diamond necklace will do nicely.

Corset: An article of clothing, often made of leather, PVC or vinyl and sometimes including strips of rigid "boning", which is tightly laced and designed to narrow the waist and lift the breasts, creating an hourglass figure.

Crop: Also called a riding crop, this is a thin, flexible instrument used for striking, consisting of a sturdy but flexible shaft wrapped with leather or a similar material, with a handle at one end and often with a small leather loop at the other.

Cuff: Any banded restraint, which may be made of metal or of a flexible material such as canvas or leather, for restricting ankles and/or wrists. Includes metal "police-style" cuffs as well as steel and leather versions with shackling rings. Don't forget to frisk.

Double-headed Dildo: Like the pushmi-pullyu, these have a head at each end so there are no fights over sharing. You can get them with the same size heads or one junior and one supersize.

Electro Sex Enhancers: A range of electro-conducive toys are available for those who like to shock their senses! These range from gloves that send a massage-like tingle to the skin, anal and urethral probes and power boxes with electrodes. Sample at your own risk.
See also Violet Wand.

Fist Mitt: Bondage/fetish gear that restrains both hands, either palm to palm or knuckles to knuckles. Also available as two separate "mittens". Both versions have rings for karabiners and cuffs.

Flogger: A tool with multiple lashes used to strike a person. Also a disciplinarian who administers flogging. Basic but effective.

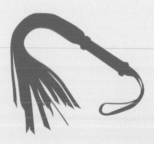

Gag: Anything used over the mouth to prevent the person from speaking or making loud sounds, or sometimes used to hold the mouth open.

Hobble Skirt: A very tight skirt that ends below the knee, which prevents freedom of motion of the legs, allowing the wearer to walk slowly in a hobbling motion. Not something you will see on the catwalk next season.

Hog Slapper: A strap of thick, heavy rubber, often wrapped in burlap or some other coarse material, for slapping when an open palm just won't do.

Hood: Any covering designed to go over the head, often partly or completely covering the face as well. Perfect for avoiding the paparazzi.

Horse: A plank supported by two legs on each end, similar to a sawhorse, for bending over and getting flogged or spanked – or practising one's trots.

Inversion Table: A flat table to which a person can be bound, and suspended between upright supports on a pivot; the table can be rotated upright, inclined, or turned completely upside-down.

Karabiner: It sounds like a type of gun but it's actually an oval or D-shaped snap link, usually with a screw lock, used by climbers and industrial riggers.

Karada: A rope harness, originating in Japan, which is tied around the torso in a series of diamond-shaped patterns. Often used as a foundation in Shibari, the Karada does not restrain the subject, and can even be worn under clothing – though perhaps it may just be easier to slip into some lingerie.

Latex: Latex, leather, rubber, vinyl, patent leather, PVC… these are all a few of a fetishist's favourite things. It's not just the skintight shiny look, but it's the feeling of being enclosed that makes these materials hands-down sexy.

Leashes & Leads: A range of leather leads to control the disobedient, including hobble belts, based on a traditional rancher's belt, that attaches to the waist, and those that clip onto collars or other binding restraints. Many suitable for use as binders and restraints.

Mouth Bit: Any of a style of gags with a long cylinder-shaped bit, usually made of soft rubber or latex, in place of a round ball. Mouth bits may include an integrated harness. Ride 'em, cowboy!

Nipple Clamp: Any device that's designed to be clamped to the nipples. May include a mechanism for adjusting or limiting the amount of pressure applied to the nipple. Clothespegs (clothespins) make good (and cheap!) nipple clamps.

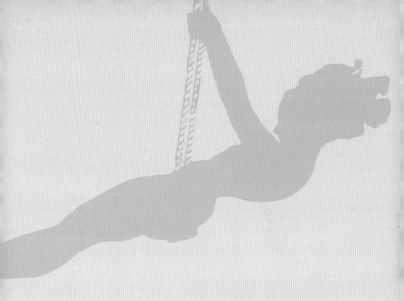

Paddle: Any stiff, hard implement, often made of wood, used for striking a person, most commonly on the rear. You never want to go up a creek without one.

Rope Cuff: Any form of tie that binds the wrists or ankles together. A knowledge of knots is a must.

Slapper: Two thick leather paddles bound together at the handle so that when a person is struck, the two paddles hit one another, creating a loud sound. No connection with getting slap happy.

Sling: Leather, canvas or nylon webbing furniture, suspended by chains or cables from the ceiling, for sit-and-swing sex.

Spanking Glove: A glove, often made of leather or heavy rubber and frequently (though not always) fingerless, designed to protect the wearer's palm as the wearer spanks another person. The bottom is up for grabs.

Speculum: These come in hand for doctor/nurse scenes. Get the right size or a bit of light roleplay could rapidly turn agonizing.

Spreader Bar: A rigid bar or rod, often with attachment points for restraints built into it at each end, designed to be attached to the feet or ankles to hold the legs spread apart. May be adjustable in length; may not be used in place of a knee press at the gym.

Straitjacket: For the ultimate restraining experience, these belted jackets – just like the trad psych-patient version – have extra-long sleeves to keep the arms pinned together at the waist. Women's versions usually expose the breasts.

Strap-on: Adjustable dildo-harness combo – both components may be bought separately!

Tickler: The keep-'em-guessing toy. You can use the soft leather strands to gently tickle your lover's curves or to deliver a quick sting across their bottom with a tiny flick of the wrist.

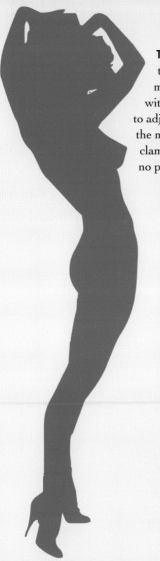

Tweezer Clamps: Long, thin, tweezer-like clamps made of flexible spring steel, with a ring that can be used to adjust their tightness. Among the mildest of all forms of nipple clamp, typically causing little or no pain.

BONDAGE & RESTRAINTS

EROTIC BONDAGE IS SO MUCH MORE THAN TYING UP SOMEONE YOU LOVE AND TANTALIZINGLY TORTURING THEM. WHAT IT'S REALLY ABOUT IS PLAYING AROUND WITH CONTROL IN YOUR LOVE PLAY - ONE OF YOU GETS TO ACT HELPLESS, THE OTHER GETS TO HAVE THEIR DELIRIOUSLY DASTARDLY WAY. DABBLING IN THESE SORTS OF POWER GAMES CAN ADD A KICK TO YOUR CARNAL CONNECTIONS - ESPECIALLY WHEN YOU'VE BEEN DOING THE SAME-OLD WITH EACH OTHER FOR A WHILE AND CRAVE SOMETHING WITH A BIT MORE SPICE THAN ORGANIZING YOURSELVES INTO A NEW PRETZEL POSITION. THE KNOWLEDGE THAT YOU CAN DO OR HAVE DONE WHAT YOU WILL (WITHIN REASON!) FOR YOUR MUTUAL MOANING PLEASURE IS MIND-BLOWING. PLUS THE TIGHT CONSTRICTION THAT

COMES WITH BEING RESTRAINED CAN BE A
SENSORY TRIP IN ITSELF, PUMPING UP ADRENALIN
AND LEADING TO MORE INTENSE, MORE BLISSFUL
- AND SIMPLY MORE - ORGASMS.

OF COURSE, THERE'S A WIDER PLAYING FIELD
IN BONDAGE THAN TYING WRISTS TO THE
BEDPOSTS. IN GENERAL THERE ARE THREE TYPES
OF BONDAGE: RESTRAINT BONDAGE, WHERE THE
GOAL IS TO RESTRICT SOMEONE'S RANGE OF
MOTION; STIMULATION BONDAGE WHERE, RATHER
THAN KEEP THEM IN CHECK, THE ROPES OR TIES
ARE THERE TO MAKE THEM WRITHE BY RUBBING
AGAINST SENSITIVE BITS OF THE BODY; AND
SUSPENSION BONDAGE - WHICH IS PRETTY MUCH
HOW IT SOUNDS - A PERSON IS BOUND FROM AN
OVERHEAD FIXTURE USING A HARNESS OR SLING
THAT WILL DANGLE THEIR ARMS, LEGS OR ENTIRE
BODY OFF THE FLOOR, ADDING A SUSPENSEFUL
EDGE OF TENSION TO THE PROCEEDINGS.

EASTERN & WESTERN
ROPE BONDAGE

These days, there are two main modes of erotic rope bondage. From the Asian shores comes the highly ritualized bondage known as Kinbaku in Japan and Shibari in the West. One of the most imaginative of all bondage styles (and arguably the most beautiful), it developed from the Japanese military restraint technique of Hojojutsu. The bondage patterns still echo the martial art with a decidedly steamy slant and are a common sight in Japanese pornography and Manga.

One of the main ways in which Shibari differs from Western bondage is that instead of knotting and wrapping the ropes to restrain and immobilize, the focus is on creating patterns. Putting knots on a person was regarded as extremely disgraceful, something some would regard as worse than death (although these days, most dabblers in Shibari will add a few knots just to finish things off). Instead, wrappings were developed that were thoughtfully designed and executed with beauty, functionality and safety in mind, to stimulate erotic pressure points such as the genitals, breasts and other hot zones. Think of it as origami, except that you're naked and folding rope instead of paper.

In contrast, in Western bondage, the emphasis is on the knot. Much of this style comes from photographer Irving Claw and artist John Willie. In their images, limbs are usually tied together (wrists, elbows, ankles, knees) and there is very little use of elaborate harnesses or instruments – and even less possibility of sex, considering the way the bodies have been bound! Instead, the erotic element comes from the predicament – such as being tied to the railroad tracks, dragged behind a horse or tied to a log at a sawmill. A damsel in distress is almost always involved.

It is probable that the uniquely human pursuit of bondage as a strictly-for-pleasure erotic endeavour actually has its roots in normal biological urges. Just watch any mammal getting it on – the male will seize the neck of the female in his teeth during mating to restrain her.

But whatever the origin, what is clear is that rather than weird and kinky, this form of sexual power play is enduringly – and endearingly – popular. Studies by sexual-desire guru Nancy Friday has found that the fantasy of being bound during intercourse is second in frequency only to the basic fantasy of getting it on with a hot babe for men, while women tend to get a warm and fuzzy feeling over the thought of being tied up and helpless to protest being ravished by some mysterious handsome dude. Bondage is clearly unbound.

TEACHING THE ROPES

Your essential all-purpose moves to becoming a bondage master. Look on www.iwillknot.com for step-by-step instructions for most common knots. Before you start, practise these two techniques until you can do them in your sleep:

1 Bight: Essentially an open loop – fold the rope in half at the middle.

2 Lark's Head: Pass the loose tails of the rope through the bight. To use it on an object (any part of the body, on furniture or a handle), wrap the rope around the object with the loop in front, and slip the tail ends through the loop from the opposite side.

Although not knots, the bight and Lark's Head will form the base of most bindings.

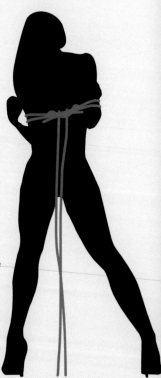

SQUARE OR REEF KNOT

This is the most commonly used knot, useful for tying packages, finishing off surgery, and your partner.

HOW TO DO IT:

If you can tie your shoes, you can make a Square knot. It's just like the first part of tying your shoes, and for the second part you repeat the first half in the opposite direction. Remember "right over left, left over right, makes a Square knot nice and tight!" Tighten by pulling the loose ends.

DON'T COME UNTIED:

If you tie right over left, right over left, you will end up with two twisted ropes known as granny knot, which isn't really much of a knot since it slips until it unties itself.

BASIC KNOTS AND BEYOND

HALF HITCH

Slightly more fiddly, this tie is best used for tying a rope to a piece of furniture such as a bedpost. It shouldn't be used on any part of the body or for suspension.

HOW TO DO IT:

Hook the rope around what you're going to bind and bring the short end under the long end, then over the top of the long end and through the space between the object and the rope. Pull tight to secure. Do two more times to create a "hitch and a half".

DON'T COME UNTIED:

It's possible for a Half Hitch to slip, but if you do three in a row, it's virtually impossible to come apart.

That's it. You are done. You now have all of the information you need to restrain your lover in pretty much any configuration your twisted little heart desires.

SHIBARI TIES

If you lean more towards the East in your bondage know-how, the fundamentals of Shibari are slightly different but still fairly simple:

1 FOLDING OR BIGHT:

You still need the bight (see page 70) – in fact, almost all Japanese rope bondage is based on this fold.

2 BANDING:

Continue to fold and refold the bight into bands or layers. The idea is that the more bands you have, the quicker you use up the rope when wrapping. Beginners should stick with one or two bands; experts can work with as much as they can handle without coming undone.

3 LAYERING:

Take several different pieces of rope or techniques and layer them on top of each other for a combo meal. For example, make a chest harness (see Karada, page 82), then taking another rope, use one of the ends to tie to the chest harness and tie the other end to a beam.

BAR WRAP

A thrifty, elegant way to use up extra rope, bar none.
Basically, you take the tails of rope and wrap them
around a band of rope nice and tight so that you end up
making a handle that you can actually grab and lift with.

HOW TO DO IT:

Loop the rope around the object you're tying to.
Hold an end in each hand. Cross the end in your right
hand over the end in your left, forming an X with your
hands and holding the pieces at the top of the X. Wrap
the end in your right hand around the object again in the
same direction as before, leaving the wrap loose. When
you bring it back around to the front, poke the end under
the piece of rope that you've just wrapped around.

DON'T COME UNTIED:

If you don't keep working your ends in the same
direction, you will end up with a knotted mess.

FRENCH BOWLINE KNOT

A good knot for binding wrists and ankles because it won't accidentally tighten and cut off circulation. You can prepare them in advance as cuffs.

HOW TO DO IT:

Lay the rope straight and then make a small loop in it, leaving a long tail. Coil the long end around the limb three or four times, each time going through the small loop. On the last trip through the loop, wrap the long end under the short end and back through the small loop in the opposite direction.

DON'T COME UNTIED:

Don't tighten as you coil – you don't want it too loose or too tight. Slide and pull the loops until they fit snugly.

BUNTLINE HITCH

A fast way to tie a rope to a fixed object such as a suspension bar or a bedpost, but not to a person because the loop tightens under tension and could restrict circulation.

HOW TO DO IT:

Loop the rope around the object (once or more). Pass the short end over the main rope segment to make a figure-of-eight, then pass it under and over the long end in a figure-of-eight in the opposite direction. Pull to tighten.

DON'T BECOME UNDONE:

Pull too soon and everything will slip.

THE PRUSIK

This is the knot you should use if you want to tighten the rope after binding, for instance, for having your Sub very tense after spread-eagling her. When not under tension, sliding the knot along the rope is easy. When tightened by the tension, it locks.

1 Make a Lark's Head (see page 70) and slip it over your partner's hand or foot so that it is around their wrist or ankle. Take the long tails and move them in the opposite direction so the loop is open and slack. The loop should be on the outside, away from the body, and the long tails on the inside, towards the body.

2 Reach through the loop and pull the long ends of the rope through. Pull on the loop again, to get some more slack, and wrap the loop around again. You may have to keep creating more slack to help the ropes move around the wrist or ankle.

3 Reach through the loop again, and pull the long ends through. Pull on the long ends, helping the ropes move around the wrist or ankle, until the wraps are comfortably snug, but not tight. Take one of the long ends and pass it under three of the wraps, starting at the outside and pulling it out the middle. Pull the end taut.

4 Take the other long end and pass it under three of the wraps, starting at the outside and pulling it out the middle. Pull the end taut. Repeat, taking one of the long ends and passing it under three of the wraps, starting at the outside and pulling it out the middle. Pull the end taut.

5 Take the other long end and pass it under three of the wraps, starting at the outside and pulling it out the middle. Pull the end taut. When your captive struggles, the loops around the wraps tighten, locking them in place so they can't tighten around the wrist or ankle.

DON'T COME UNTIED:
Be careful not to make the wraps too tight to begin with. You don't need to; they are secure even if they are only fairly snug, and if you make them too tight, you will cut off circulation.

FIGURE EIGHT KNOT

A nice smooth knot used as an ending for a rope
– stopping it from slipping inside a hole or ring or
preventing unravelling.

HOW TO DO IT:

Form a figure-of-eight with the end of the rope, passing
the short end through the first loop. Pull to tighten.

DON'T COME UNTIED:

Make sure the rope is thick so the knot doesn't just slip
through the ring or hole.

CROSSED LIMBS BINDING

Use when you want to tie your partner's hands at the
back or front or to tie the ankles with the knees apart.

HOW TO DO IT:

Rest the centre of the rope against their crossed limbs.
Coil the rope around the limbs three or four times.
Cross the ends of the rope. The one that will go down
passes over the one that will go up. This step is needed
to change the direction on the rope without pinching or
putting undue pressure on the limbs. Then coil a couple
of times up and down, passing the rope between the limbs
vertically. Finally, finish the binding by tying both ends of
the rope with a Square knot (see page 71).

Check that you can pass at least a finger between the
ropes and the skin. If you can't, loosen the binding and
next time, don't make the coils so tight.

CROSSED LIMBS BINDING

Use when you want to tie your partner's hands at the
back or front or to tie the ankles with the knees apart.

HOW TO DO IT:

Rest the centre of the rope against their crossed limbs.
Coil the rope around the limbs three or four times.
Cross the ends of the rope. The one that will go down
passes over the one that will go up. This step is needed
to change the direction on the rope without pinching or
putting undue pressure on the limbs. Then coil a couple
of times up and down, passing the rope between the limbs
vertically. Finally, finish the binding by tying both ends of
the rope with a Square knot (see page 71).

DON'T COME UNTIED:

Check that you can pass at least a finger between the
ropes and the skin. If you can't, loosen the binding and
next time, don't make the coils so tight.

PARALLEL LIMBS BINDING
(TWO-COLUMN TIE)

Ties the ankles or wrists so that the arms or knees are
pulled tightly together.

HOW TO DO IT:

Lay the centre of the rope across your partner's limbs
and coil it three or four times around both limbs. When
the coils are finished, cross the ropes, the one going down
over the one going up, as above. Secure things with a
couple of vertical coils crossways and finish
with a Square knot.

DON'T COME UNTIED:

It's the horizontal/vertical hatching that gives this tie its
strength so don't pull it too tight while coiling. Make sure
you can pass the finger test, slipping one finger between
the rope and the skin.

PRETZEL HOGTIE

This is the most strenuous restraint you can do without
actually tying someone down. Gag and/or blindfold
your bottom. The wrists are hogtied back tightly to the
ankles or knee ropes. A shoulder harness is then secured
to the ankle ropes and pulled until the spine bends back.
Then the big toes are tied together, and the gag or the
blindfold is leashed back to the big toes and pulled until
the head and neck are arched back. Schedule a trip to
the physical therapist.

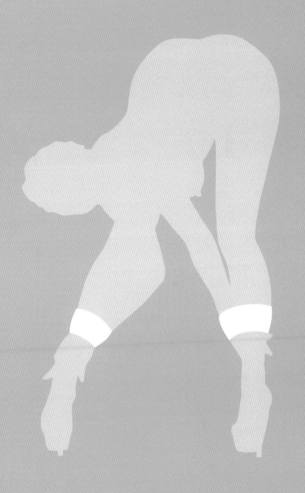

NO KNOTS

If you're all thumbs when it comes to tying knots, don't despair. You can still indulge in some restraint play without getting all bound up. These wraps and devices don't include a single tie.

KARADA

An easy form of Shibari, this rope harness can be tied in about 15 minutes, and there's not a single knot in it.

1 Start with an extra-long 15 m (50 ft) rope to leave lots of rope for some bells and whistles once you're done. Make a bight so it drapes around the back of the person's neck with the tails draping down the front of the body.

2 Bring the ends of the rope around one another three times – these three twists will become the three diamonds you see in the front of the finished rope harness. Bring the two ends of the rope between your partner's legs, then up and apart on the other side.

3 From this point, each end of the rope will wrap around their hips and then through the lowest twist in front, which is much easier to do than to read about… See? Nothing to it.

4 Don't pull the rope tight; as you continue this process, bringing the ends of the rope around to the front, passing them through the twists, and then bringing them back again, the rope will need to slide to let the diamonds open up in the front. It's okay if the rope is loose at this point; it will become tighter as you work your way up. Repeat two more times.

5 After the last twist, bring the ends of the rope over the shoulder tops or back around beneath their arms so that the rope goes around to the front of their body, through the topmost twist, then back around behind them again. Now bring the ends up underneath the rope where it passes around the neck, and down beneath the rope, wrapping around their back. (Again, easier than it sounds.)

6 You can tie off or tuck in the ends of the rope wherever you like – around the part where it loops around the back of the neck, or around the part where it crosses behind their back – but that would be a waste of a good rope. Instead, segue into a Frog Tie – see page 84.

FROG TIE

1 Tell your partner to kneel. Take the leftover rope and bring it down between your partner's legs. Then pass it under and up around the leg, and keep wrapping around the person's leg a few times so that it is snug but not tight.

2 Bring it between their upper and lower leg, pass it around all the wrappings and back between their upper and lower leg again. At this point, you'll adjust how tight the wrappings are around the leg – the tighter you pull the loop of rope around the wrappings, the tighter they'll be.

3 From there, take the end of the rope up along the person's inner thigh. Almost done – just take whatever amount of rope is left at the end and wrap it around and around the lower part of the Karada where it comes across their bottom. When you've reached the end, just tuck the last bit of rope underneath the wrap.

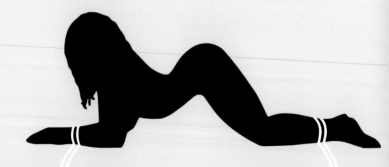

CHAIN HARNESS

You can also make a Karada out of chain. The chain should have openable links because it won't wrap or tie like rope.

1 Start with a 10 m (33 ft) length of chain, find the bight and slip it over your partner's head so that it hangs down the front of their body.

2 Twist the chain and hold the twisted sections open to create diamonds in the front (command your partner to hold the chain or you may lose the diamond).

3 Bring the ends down between their legs, then up behind them, around their body, and through the section in front.

4 Repeat until you reach the top, then bring it over their shoulders and down their back. Use a chain link that can be opened, a small padlock or carabineer to link the chain together behind their neck.

5 Take the excess length of chain and tuck it beneath the chain, passing around the body. You can secure them to a fixed object or leave it hanging like a tail between their legs.

BARS & CUFFS

Besides good old-fashioned rope, there's lots of other tools to bind up your lover, from tape and leather cuffs to chains and spreader bars. Here's a run-down on how to use the favourites.

UNDER-THE-BED RESTRAINTS

Skip the complicated hardware. This simple, discreet cuff set, made to stay in place in your bed with a connector slide, renders your lover helpless in a snap. Available from good sex shops (try www.lovehoney.co.uk or www.amazon.com), they are particularly useful for those who have beds without bedposts, as the straps are anchored under the mattress and can be positioned in various ways. They can also be linked together end-to-end and worn as a collar or thigh cuff.

> **Warning:** Zip ties hold the tie well but are almost impossible to remove and can cut into flesh, while electrical cord can't hold the knot well, no matter how much of an extra electrical charge it gets. Don't use these!

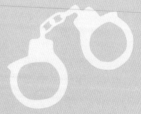

CUFFS

Considered an "entry level" restraint, cuffs for the ankles and wrists often have D-rings or locking mechanisms for attaching to spreader bars, chains and ropes as well as to each other. Use four together to tie wrists to ankles in a hogtie. They can also be combined with belts or tape to form a ball tie, where the subject is bend double into a ball with the heels against the buttocks and the arms hugging the legs.

SPREADER BARS

This rigid metal or wooden bar with cuffs on both ends is designed to keep the arms or legs wide apart and immobilized, providing unimpeded access to the body. A pair of them keeps the person spread-eagled and if If bars are attached between the knees and ankles, the subject can only walk with bent knees. The bars, which have attachment points along their length for collars or anchoring ropes, chains and karabiners, can be anchored to a bed, the floor, walls or the ceiling for suspension play.

Warning: Not all spreader bars are designed to support the weight of the human body!

SUSPENSION

Suspension is any form of bondage in which the person bound is hanging partially or completely off the floor, often by ropes affixed to an overhead point or by means of a rigid bar with attached suspension cuffs. For serious bondage players only.

Almost any suspension is going to cause at least medium discomfort. Put a short (as in 15 minutes max) time limit or use a full-support suspension such as a swing, sling or thigh-straps to support the weight of the body to avoid the suspension damaging your body. Tie the wrists and ankles where and how you desire. You'll need some sort of suspension bar to hang from. And definitely invest in a panic snap, which is designed to be able to be opened even under high tension by sliding a spring-loaded metal collar upward.

PREDICAMENT BONDAGE

This is a type of bondage in which the intent is to place the bound person in an awkward, difficult, inconvenient or uncomfortable situation, or to set out a challenge for the bound person to overcome. For example, a person might be bound in such a way that their hands and feet are mostly but not completely immobilized, then asked to perform a task (such as to serve their lover a drink or make dinner).

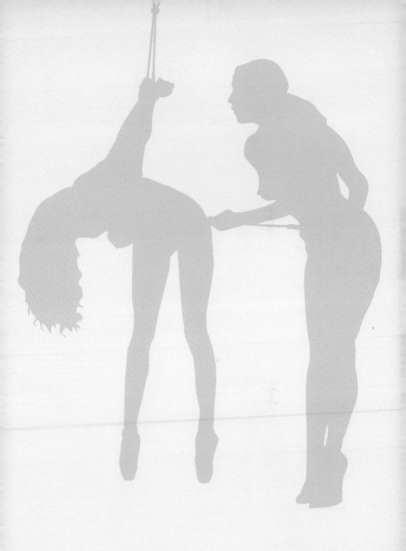

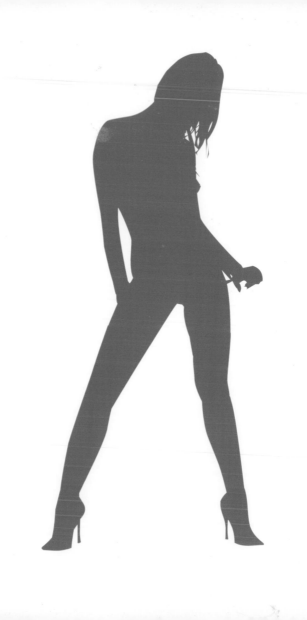

HAIR BONDAGE

W̲hile you don't need to be a trained stylist, you should feel comfortable tying knots – working your tresses into your power play can be fussy, as it is easy to brush up against accidental scalping if you tie too tight. Apart from the feeling it gives of being restrained, it also makes for handy control to keep the head still and in position for "forced" oral sex.

Skip the headache if you have short hair. It won't work. But if your locks are shoulder-length or longer, gather the hair in a loose ponytail at the back centre of the head and give it a spritz of hairspray. This will make the hair less slippery so it will stick to the rope and to itself.

This is one time you want to make your knots and pulls as tight as possible.

THE RING

This may work on slightly shorter hair (you'll need a high frustration threshold) and it's a good beginner tie. Take a strand of hair, lead it through a ring (any kind of ring will do, such as those found in hardware and DIY shops) and fold it around it. Make sure the part between the head and the ring is one-third of the hair and the part that's folded back is two-thirds. Wrap either thin packing rope or fishing line around the folded strand, starting from the ring and working towards the head. When finished, fold the remaining one-third upwards and repeat the wrapping, this time up towards the ring. Tie the rope with a Square knot (see page 71). Now the ring can be used as a connection point for any other bondage (the possibilities are endless: from tying the Sub's hands behind their head to fastening the ring to a wall hook or a quick snap-hook to link it to handcuffs).

JAPANESE BRAIDING

Japanese bondage masters prefer special rice rope for this, but hemp's rough surface will do just as well. You'll need time to work this intricate method, but the good news is that once tied correctly, it can be kept in for days and used for a wide variety of moves. Take three or four thin ropes and bunch them together as one rope. Lay the middle of the bundle behind the ponytail and wrap both ends around the tail two or three times, about one third of the length of the ponytail from the head. Next divide both the rope bundle and the hair into three strands and plait (braid) them again, going down as far as you can. When done, separate the rope from the hair and tie the rope strings together with a series of Square knots (see page 71). You can now either use the remainder of the rope bundle (if long enough) to tie it to something else or tie another rope to the end of the braided bundle to use in the rest of your bondage.

THE KNOT TUBE

Again, break out the hemp rope. Separate a strand of hair (or use an entire ponytail) and work from the middle of the rope. Wrap it around the strand close to the head once and make a Square knot (see page 71), stopping halfway. Now lay the strand of hair over the knot and make another half reef knot. Wrap the rope around the strand again and repeat the procedure. Repeat this over and over again.

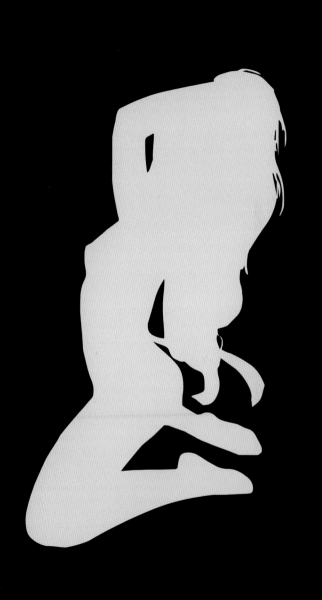

BREAST BONDAGE

Most commonly using rope to bind the naked breasts, this form of bondage can also be achieved using webbing straps or a harness – see also Karada, the Japanese version of the rope harness, on page 82. Breast bondage can be combined with other techniques and used for attaching to other props or bindings and applied over clothing or directly to the skin, worn under clothing or in full view.

Breast punishment, in the form of nipple clamps, flogging, biting and scratching date as far back as the Kama Sutra, and bondage allows the breasts to be up front and centre for some serious handling. There are different forms:

Circling: Using a rope, ribbon or leather thong, each breast is wrapped with two turns around the base and secured with a square knot. The ends can be run together in the front to tie the breasts closer together or behind the back to lift and separate.

Rope "Bra": In this type, the rope is wrapped under her breast, high on the ribcage, then between the breasts and finally above the breasts and under the arms, knotted in the back. The breast will be accentuated and surrounded by the ropes, but no pressure is applied directly.

Breast Binder: In this, the breasts are squashed against the chest, to make them smaller. Best achieved with a bandage-style wrap, begin by wrapping under the breast at the ribcage, then wrap above the breasts and work downwards to completely cover. Finish off at the back.

◇ **Warning: Take care in this area, and go lightly.**
◇ **Breasts can be very delicate and vulnerable and**
◇ **hard or deep strikes or prolonged binding can**
◇ **damage the tissue.**

BOOB TREATMENTS

TO FLATTEN:
Bondage tape, ace bandages, plastic wraps

TO TEASE:
Ice cubes, nipple clamps, feathers

TO TORTURE:
Paddle, spanking, nibbling, scratching

TO RESTRAIN:
Nipple clamps, tight corset

BONDAGE GLOSSARY

Ball Tie: A specific form of bondage in which the person is bound in a seated position with the knees up, the head bent down over the knees, and the hands behind the back. This posture is for the strong of heart only as it quickly becomes extremely fatiguing.

Bend: A knot that binds the ends of two ropes together. Also what you need to do if you want to incorporate a little S&M-lite into your play.

Bight: A rope folded back on itself to form a narrow loop.

Binding: A knot that restricts object(s) by making multiple winds.

Box Tie: A specific form of bondage in which a person brings their arms together, grips each forearm with the opposite hand, and then ropes are wound around them. Talk about being tightly wound!

Breaking Strength: The manufacturer's estimation of the load a rope (on new rope without knots or kinks) will bear before it ruptures.

Crossing Turn: A circle of rope made with the rope crossing itself. This has nothing to do with changing your mind mid-tie.

Cock Bondage: Tying or restraining the penis. Or marriage for some men.

Frapping Turns: Additional turns made at right angles in lashings, whippings and seizings to tighten the main turns. Also the way someone dances after too many beers.

Frog Tie: A specific form of bondage in which the person kneels and the ankles are bound to the thighs, preventing the person from rising; the wrists are then bound to the ankles. Kiss and you may turn your frog into a prince(ss).

Grommet: A continuous circle of rope. Also known as a sling. If you want to really mess with their minds, challenge your lover to find the beginning.

Half Hitch: A crossing turn, often made round a part of the body or an object. The crossing holds the lower part in place.

Hogtie: When the ankles and wrists are bound together, usually behind the back; then the ankles are tied to the wrists while the person lies on his or her stomach.

Jam: When a knot cannot be untied readily. In other words, you have a hitch.

Kami: Any technique that involves the hair, such as weaving ropes through the hair to hold the head immobile.

Karada: a rope harness, originating in Japan, which is tied around the torso in a series of diamond-shaped patterns. Often used as a foundation in Shibari, the Karada does not restrain the subject, and can even be worn under clothing – though perhaps it may just be easier to slip into some lingerie.

Kink: A tight turn in a rope that can form during use and may damage rope fibres. Also how bondage is often described.

Knot: The generic word for all rope and cordage tucks and ties.

Kotori: A rope harness intended to support a person's weight from the torso and upper legs. Chopsticks not included.

Laid Rope: Rope made by twisting. And it's very happy.

Lashing: A knot usually used to hold poles together. But may also be what your lover wants to give you.

Lay: The direction of the twist in the rope away from the viewer, either clockwise (right-handed, Z laid) or anticlockwise (left-handed, S laid).

Line: Another word for rope, but generally small cordage of less than 12.5 mm (½ in) in diameter. Might also be something handed to you in order to get you in a compromising position.

Loop: A knot used to create a closed circle in a line.

One-Column Tie: In bondage, any form of tie that binds one part of the body to something else – such as the arm to the headboard.

Psychological Bondage: Bondage without the use of ropes or other restraints. It's all in the voice command.

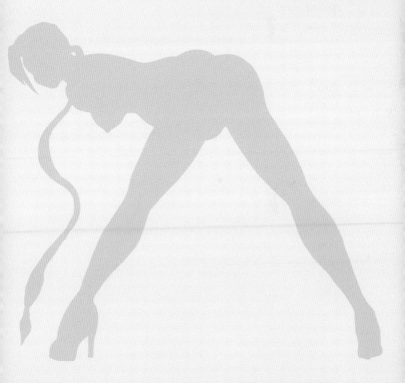

Rope Cuff: Any form of tie that binds the wrists or ankles together. A knowledge of knots is a must.

Rope Splice: A knot formed by interweaving strands of rope rather than whole lines. More time consuming to do, but usually stronger than simple knots and you don't need a ring.

Round Turn: When a rope is wrapped so that it passes around the back of a body part or object twice. If you can follow that, you will have no trouble making strong rope splices.

Running End: Also called the "working end", refers to the tip of the rope that forms a knot, and not what you do once you have trussed up your lover.

Seize: To join two ropes or parts of ropes together with a binding of small cordage. May also refer to what you will want to do to your partner if they lose the key to the handcuffs.

Self-Bondage: Tying one's self up or otherwise restraining one's self, sometimes as a part of masturbation. Often tricky and always lonely.

Shibari: A type of bondage originating in Japan and characterized by extremely elaborate patterns of rope, often used both to restrain and to stimulate by binding or compressing breasts and/or genitals.

Shinju: A type of Japanese rope harness that goes around and over the breasts. A shinju does not restrict motion and can be worn under clothing; as the subject moves, the ropes shift against the breasts, providing constant stimulation. Aramaa!

Spread Eagle: Wrists and ankles are tied to bedposts, a door frame or other anchoring devices so that the limbs are splayed out.

Sukaranbo/ Sukuranbo: A type of rope harness that wraps around the buttocks and upper thighs and passes between the legs and over the genitals, passing between the lower lips of a female wearer. The rope may feature a knot at the place where it touches the clitoris.

Takatekote: A type of rope harness, originating in Japan, which goes around the torso and holds the arms behind the back.

Two-Column Tie: Like the single except two parts of the body are tied together.

DISCIPLINE &
PUNISHMENT

IN BDSM, PUNISHMENT IS A TOOL TO CORRECT
WRONGDOING OR LACK OF ACTION BUT IT
DOESN'T NECESSARILY INVOLVE PAIN. RESTRICTIVE
MOVEMENT OR BONDAGE, HUMILIATION, VERBAL
"DRESSING DOWN" OR EVEN JUST A LOOK CAN
WORK – IT ALL DEPENDS ON THE INDIVIDUAL
INVOLVED AS SOME FORMS OF PUNISHMENT ARE
OTHER PEOPLE'S REWARDS. TYPICAL PUNISHMENTS
ARE SPANKING, CANING OR EVEN GENITORTURE,
BUT FOR THE BEGINNER, THIS IS BEST EXPLORED
IN A ROLEPLAY SITUATION AS "PLAY PUNISHMENT"
RATHER THAN THE REAL KIND. LUCKILY,
PUNISHMENT IS ALWAYS FOLLOWED BY REWARD
(THE ORGASM!) IN POWER PLAY.

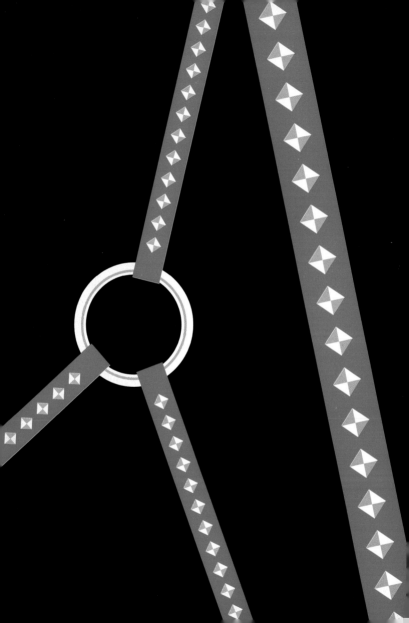

CANING IT

These tips may help you decide what to use to pack a wallop.

Ticklers are sticks with feathers at the end. A leather tickler is a keep-'em-guessing toy – you can use the soft leather strands to gently tickle your lover's curves – or to deliver a quick sting across their bottom with a tiny flick of the wrist.

A crop is a small (usually leather) whip. Some crops come with a narrow flat "flapper" on one end of a flexible shaft for that oh-so-sexy tickle/whip combo. All you need is a flick of the wrist to power one.

Canes come in a wide variety from the domestic (usually straight and made from bamboo) to the schoolmaster's cane (a curved handle and more traditional). Novice spankers should work with shorter equipment – no longer than 1 m (3 ft) – to hone their accuracy and speed. Thicker canes cut the skin less often but cause more bruising. Thin canes cause more of a stinging feeling than the thud effect of their larger counterparts. It's your choice.

A switch is simply a cane that has been split at the bottom end to produce a fork or two tongues.

Floggers: The word "flogging" may conjure up images of pirates punishing scallywags bound to the mizzenmast – which is one way to get into some scrummy roleplay. Basically, a flogger is any whipping device with a number of leather "tails" or falls tied together to a handle, which is covered with braided leather. There are lots of variations, but the important differences are the type and weight of the leather used for the tails, and how their tips are shaped. Deerskin leather, for example, is very light and soft, making it almost impossible to do much, if any, injury, while bison and bull leather are heavy duty. The most common flogger is the cat-o-nine tails; its nine tails are often braided and end in a plain or knotted tip.

Whips: These are anything with one tail. Real ones can inflict pretty serious damage and are best left to the experts – like bronco busters. If you really want to beat it, try a specially made kind that doesn't hurt no matter how hard it's swung. Some – like one called the "Latex Whip on a Stick" – even sound painful when they come into contact with the skin, but are more likely to make you sigh than cry. Foam rounders or baseball bats also guarantee a soft, satisfying landing.

Spanking paddle: You'll be belting out "Hurts So Good" when your lover gives you a smackdown. There are some scary-looking paddles available (spikes, anyone?) so save your money and use a ping-pong racquet instead. Mix pleasure with the pain by pausing between spankings and massaging their bottom with your hands.

BEGINNER'S TOOLS

Start out with a small paddle or riding crop, which is easy to guide and more accurate than a flogger or whip. You won't lose your power punch – even lightweight ones can make it uncomfortable for someone to sit down for days.

A slapper has a flat (usually leather) surface with another, hinged flap of leather attached to it so that it makes an extra loud noise upon impact – think sexy sound effects. Some are lined with fleece on the receiving end to cushion the blow. They're small, so you can easily carry one for whenever and wherever the impulse strikes.

WHAT A SPANKER!

Spanking and fantasy are the dynamic duo of the BDSM scene. Experienced spankers concentrate on the mental foreplay first by announcing the "punishment" and ordering their 'badly behaved' partner to stand in the corner and wait for punishment. Favourite plays include daddy or uncle and naughty girl, teacher and badly behaved student, and so on. End with a bang – the receiver promises to mend their ways and shows just how good they can be.

Up for some playful paddling? Here are some sizzling ways to have a spanking good time.

1 However you sock it to 'em – hand, paddle, hairbrush – start off striking lightly, then gradually make the beat more intense. If you hit too strong too soon and too quickly, you will hurt your lover in a definitely not sexy way.

2 It is the quantity of slaps that does the trick, not so much the impact and force. Their bottom is not your boss's face, so don't smash it to a pulp. Start by rubbing it – you can rub one or both cheeks – and then you should smack only one cheek at a time. Don't worry, before you know it, they'll turn the other cheek...

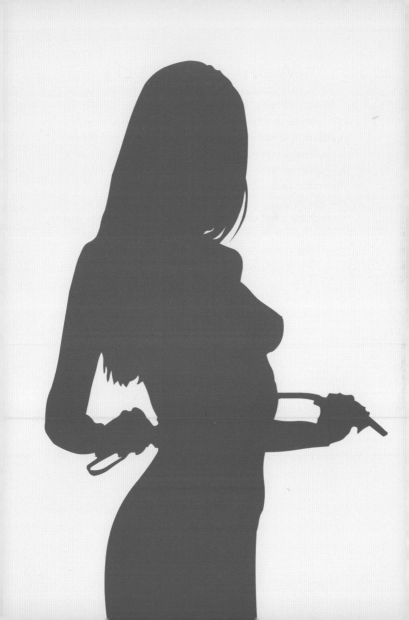

3 The further your hips are bent, the stronger the impact. So it's better to strike a pose over on your hands and knees, over your lover's lap, the kitchen table, the bonnet (hood) of your car – use your imagination. The classic pose lets you brace yourself against their blows while exposing your rear for a good licking.

4 The key to making your smackdown blissful is location, location, location. Hit the bull's-eye by aiming where the butt cheek meets the thigh, or spread the buns and softly spank the anal area with two or three fingers. Spanking close to the genitals will also send the receiver into sweet oblivion.

5 To intensify things, don't hit harder. Instead, relax your wrist. If you're using your hand, alternate between spreading your fingers to widen the stingy effect and cupping your hands to smooth things over. Take a breather after each smack to let the sensation sink in. Mix the moment up with a bottom rub before resuming. For a wildly wanton whack, spank with a leather-gloved hand.

6 Work some light stroking, scratching, and rubbing into your spanking. Don't forget to rub-a-dub-dub their other bits and pieces at the same time to keep things painfully fabulous. If you're using a hairbrush, switch things around and use the bristle side every few smacks.

7 Good spankers have good rhythm. The winning beat is: two light smacks, one slightly harder, then three light smacks and one hard one, and repeat. This build-up will deem you master.

GLOSSARY

Over the Knee (OTK): A style of spanking which is pretty much what it sounds like. Bottom's up.

Impact Play: Anything involving striking or hitting – for example flogging, spanking, percussion or whipping.

Percussion: Any form of impact play involving striking with a blunt or fairly heavy implement – such as a buck hammer or bass drum.

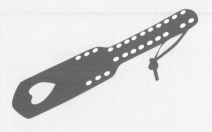

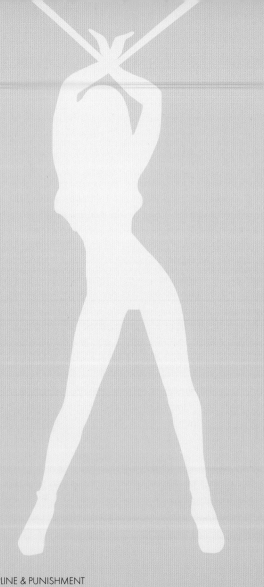

GENITORTURE

There are many forms of genitorture (the name says it all), such as clamps, clips, forceps, leather thongs, massage bongers, ropes, silk, spoons, weights and whips, but it can also simply be done with the hands, tongue and mouth. However more intense scenes require the right tools.

The psychological effect can be huge because the punishment concentrates on the genitals, the most delicate and vulnerable area of the body.

CLAMPS AND CLIPS

Clamps are pretty much what they sound like: devices used for gripping onto various body parts such as nipples, balls and vaginal lips. Some nipple clamps are designed to simply give a light nip or a pull. Some are designed to produce a heavy pinch. And some actually have teeth on them that do a biting thing. The crème de la crème are vibrating clamps that give a full-body pinch and buzz. Nipple-to-vulva/penis clamps (Y clamps) connect all of your best bits. There are alligator (not recommended for the novice as they are fairly fierce), tweezer (delicate and rubber-tipped), bull-nose (with screws for tightening) and clover (Japanese "butterfly" type) too.

Clips are small devices that grip onto different areas of the body, like BDSM bling for the clitoris, nipples, labia and penis. They usually come in heavy metals like gold and silver, and may be topped with rhinestones and – sigh – mini vibrators.

NIPPLE CLAMP TIPS

- Ensure the nipple is erect before placing clamps on.

- Don't leave them on for more than 10-15 minutes.

- Gently tug or brush the clamps for increased sensation.

- Try to find adjustable versions so you can set them to pinch harder or softer.

- Start by clamping as much flesh as possible and adjust to less to increase the pressure and sensation.

- Coldness, numbness, and discoloration are signals that it is time to release the clamp.

Warning: Test the clamp on the wrist or less sensitive piece of skin before using it on a sensitive area. Don't leave clamps on for long until you see how much your partner enjoys it – too much of any one kind of stimulation can become annoying.

SMALL WHIPS

Specially made whips for the intimate female genitals are available, and these are shorter and lighter and often found in leather, suede, plastic and rubber. They still deliver a light sting, but with less impact. Don't use anything too hard or thuddy. Light slapping with the hand can deliver just the right "wowza" reaction.

COCK AND BULL

Cock restraints, weights and cages are all part and parcel of CBT (cock and bull torture). Like with women, you don't want to use heavy canes or paddles. One of the most impressive devices is, without question, the ball crusher. A handsome, heavy chunk of gleaming metal machinery, the base of the ball crusher locks snugly around the testicles, then wing nuts tighten a metal bar securely against them. The testicles are pressed flat – or as flat as they'll go without popping. Picture two rolling pins coming together, mashing the balls. Ouch.

If you want to play it down, you can squeeze, knead, push, pull, massage and slap the genital area. The mix of pleasure and pain is sure to drive him crazy!

SENSATION
PLAY

SENSITIZE YOUR LOVEMAKING WITH THE SWEET
SIDE OF POWER GAMES. SENSATION PLAY RELATES
TO ANY ACTIVITY THAT ADDS OR MODIFIES
SENSATIONS, OR INDEED DIMINISHES OR DEPRIVES
YOU OF THEM. RUBBING, TICKLING, STROKING,
LICKING, BITING AND SCRATCHING CAN CREATE
A MIND-BENDING EXPERIENCE AND RELEASE
PLEASURABLE ENDORPHINS.

OFTEN UNDERTAKEN BLINDFOLDED, YOUR PARTNER
IS TOTALLY IN CONTROL OVER WHAT YOU ARE
FEELING AND WHEN, CREATING A SENSORY
OVERLOAD THAT CAN ENHANCE ALMOST EVERY
OTHER SEXUAL ACTIVITY. BLINDFOLDS AND
RESTRAINTS ARE USED TO PREVENT THE SUBJECT
FROM TAKING CONTROL OVER WHAT THEY ARE
EXPERIENCING, SO IT IS A GREAT WAY TO FIRST
INTRODUCE BONDAGE INTO YOUR LOVEMAKING.

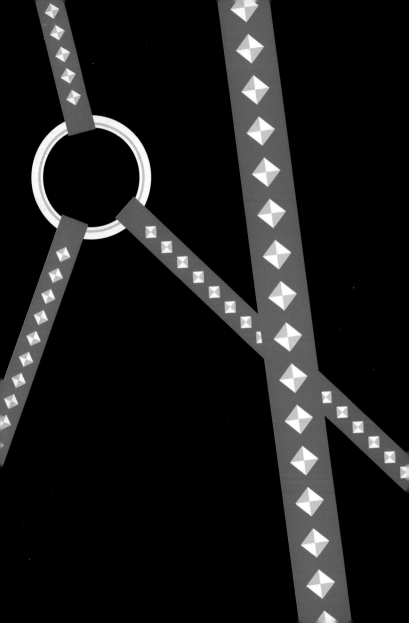

THE FIVE SENSES

Take your time and explore your five senses with these suggestions.

TOUCH

- Roll a Wartenberg wheel across the skin, varying the pressure.

- Stroke or tickle with feathers.

- Run velvet, silk or other soft cloth over the breasts and genitals.

- Rub coarse material, such as sandpaper, hessian or canvas, on the naked skin.

- Try hot and cold play (see Wax play, page 120).

- Blow hot or cold air over your partner's body using a hairdryer or fan.

- Trace ice cubes slowly over the bare skin, breasts and nipples, as well as into the hollow of the throat and inner thighs.

- Make a popsicle dildo and watch it melt!

- Chill or heat a metal beaded-chain flogger and draw across the skin.

- Put on a "vampire glove". Made of teethed leather, this can be used to stroke gently or more aggressively.

TASTE

- Feed your partner something especially hot, cold, sweet or spicy.

- Spoon semen between her lips.

- Squeeze something unpleasant, like lemon juice, into the mouth.

- Have a food feast on your partner's body - nyotaimori is the Japanese ritual of eating sushi off a naked person.

- Crunch up some mints before oral play.

- Get gloopy with splosh - www.splosh.com - and turn your body into a delicious delight.

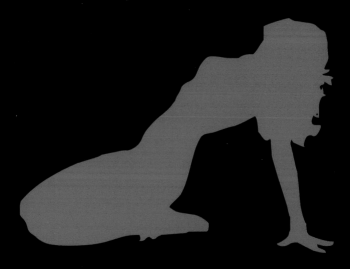

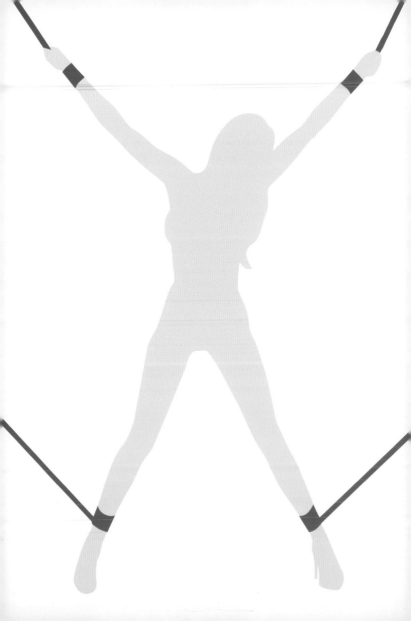

HEARING

- Turn up the volume and pump up the bass.

- Vary the music from soft and gentle to rocking.

- Use a metronome or play tapping sounds.

- Play threatening sounds like loud crashes, screams
  or thuds of a paddle.

- Script some dirty talking and subject your subject to
  a lashing of your tongue.

SMELL

- Overwhelm the sense of smell with something
  like ammonia or vinegar.

- Spray perfumes or relaxing herbal scents nearby.

- Use food odours, particularly if your subject is hungry.

SIGHT

- Turn on flashing lights or strobes.

- Turn the lights down, then up – play with extremes.

WAX PLAY

Full-scale users cover themselves head-to-toe in a polished waxsuit, but all you need are a few melted drops to heat up your homefires. Play with temperatures. Alternate between hot wax and ice for extremes that will drive your sweetie wild, or use a blindfold.

To get the more sensitive bits of the body like the nipples and family jewels in on the action with all of the pleasure and none of the pain, run your finger along the edge of the candle so you get a wax-covered finger. Then let that finger stroke and poke where it will.

Smear your ride in edible massage wax, and then polish their fenders with your tongue.

HEAT THINGS UP WITH WAX

Put your partner in a horizontal position (it makes it much easier to drip wax onto them). Have some ice cubes handy to cool their skin. If they're into the pain as well as the pleasure, scrape off the wax with your fingernails afterwards.

HOT WAX TIPS

- Cheap, unscented white candles work better than the perfumed, coloured beeswax kinds because they burn more slowly. Tilt the candle slightly so the hot wax drops one drip at a time.

- If he's a fuzzy wuzzy bear, he should shave first or plan to spend the rest of his life picking wax chunks off his body.

- Oiling the skin before waxing makes removal easier later. Massage oils seem to stay cooler than baby oil, which gets hot under wax.

- Be very careful about lingerie, as some items will melt or burn, sticking to the skin and causing serious burns. Avoid nylon, vinyl, PVC and patent leather.

FEED THE KITTY

Here 8 wall-shaking, earth-quaking sensational moves
that'll make your partner end up across the room (you
might want to tie them down, too).

Use one or all. Think of them as your must-do list of
starter techniques to tie, sigh, tease, squeeze and totally
please. Be prepared – they'll beg you give them relief
(and isn't that the idea?). If you're feeling particularly
evil, don't offer any relief at all! But definitely take your
turn – when you're ready, straddle (face or groin – you
get to choose) and instruct them on exactly how to bring
you pleasure.

MUTE IT

Cover their ears with ear muffs, earphones hooked into
music (your choice if you make it something they
love or hate) – anything that restricts hearing so
they can concentrate on how their other senses
are being tortured.
Up the amps with
an OhMiBod
music-powered
vibrator.

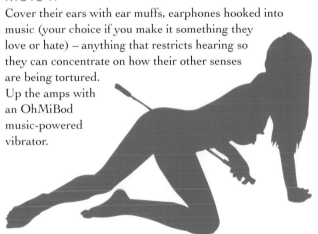

BE BREAST IN SHOW

When they're all wrapped up with no place to go, you can:

- Add a cold chill to your play by wrapping the breasts in chains that have been stored in the freezer.

- Pinch an inch. Nipples can be some of the most sensitive bits on the human body – his and hers. You can buy nipple clamps, vibroclips and tweezers that adjust to add just the right squeeze, but clothespegs (clothespins) and rubberbands are good emergency subs. Don't leave them on for more than 15 minutes at a time. Don't worry that it's not long enough – the really exquisite ache starts when the pressure is released.

- Drip warm wax around the exposed flesh of breasts wrapped in a chest harness (see Karada page 82).

- Crank up the heat by alternating with an ice cube rub.

MAKE SURPRISE MOVES

When you're making your way up your partner's body, be it with kisses or with drizzled syrup, going in a straight line doesn't work as effectively as zig-zagging. Nerves like surprises, and if you're working in a straight line, the body knows what's coming next.

USE YOUR MOUTH

Bondage without oral should simply be considered wrong. Bondage with straight-through-to-orgasm oral should also be considered wrong. But bondage with teasing, tantalizing oral – oo la la! Kiss and suck and bite them all over, then return again to some straight oral play. Toy with them manually. Change gears as often as you're able.

JUST ADD WATER

…Or lube, as the case may be. When liquid combines with bondage, you get awesome surface tension.

ADD PAIN TO PLEASURE

This isn't about drawing blood (unless you want to). But bondage and spanking or smacking with a whip or paddle go together. As a rule, strokes from whips and paddles are delivered to fleshy, muscled body areas such as the lower buttocks and the "lower half of the upper half" of the back. But you can also use a nylon rope flogger that's been frayed out, a ribbon flogger made of thin strands of satin ribbon or a rubber duster whip made of thin rubber strings about the size of angel-hair pasta, which let you whack away without the pain (no matter how hard you hit).

◇ **WARNING:** It's very dangerous to strike kidneys,
◇ liver, spleen or tailbone.

7 TICKLE

Watch them wiggle and squirm. Use your fingers or, better yet, a feather (there are specific ticklers made for the purpose available from sex shops). Run it up the small of the back and below the buttocks for a totally tantalizing sensation.

USE HOUSEHOLD OBJECTS

Your house is chockablock with gear. Try dragging the prongs of a fresh-from-the-freezer ice-cold fork up the inside of their leg, or teasing their privates with the bristles of a silicone pastry brush. Use a curtain tassel to tease and tickle. Even a piece of paper being dragged up a naked body will make them shiver. A comb or brush, body lotion, a paintbrush: anything works, provided you begin with light pressure and see what the reaction is.

RESOURCES

Ann Summers
For sex toys, costumes, kits and erotica
www.annsummers.com

Babeland
Babe-friendly sex and bondage toys
www.babeland.com

B E S T Slave Training
How-tos for bondage knots and hitches
www.bestslavetraining.com/Bondageknot.htm

Blowfish
Bondage tips and pointers, handbooks and gear
www.blowfish.com/catalog/guides/

Bondage Gear
Hoods, whips, gags, rope and restraints, delivered in discreet packaging
www.bondagegear.co.uk

Coco de Mer
Luxury top-quality bondage gear, such as silver cuffs and collars, leather reins and harnesses, corsets, masks and rope
www.coco-de-mer.com/shop/bondage

Deviants Dictionary
An online guide to bondage terms and knots
public.diversity.org.uk/deviant/ssknots.htm

Extreme Restraints
Quality bondage and fetish gear including furniture, suspension equipment and sleepsacks
www.extremerestraints.com

Good Vibrations
An online sex superstore providing all kinds of bondage and fetish toys, harnesses and strap-ons
www.goodvibrations.com

Libida
Offers harnesses,
restraints and other toys,
as well as erotica
www.libida.com

Love Honey
Vibrators, gifts, whips
and more: the online
orgasm superstore
www.lovehoney.co.uk

OhMiBod
Hi-tech sex toys that
connect to mobile phones
and other sockets
www.ohmibod.com

The Pleasure Chest
A treasure trove of
pleasure devices with
a BDSM section
www.thepleasurechest.
com

Simply Pleasure
A climactic collection of
tools, including whips,
bondage and fetish
www.simplypleasure.com

Stockroom
Quality sex toys, bondage
gear, restraints, chastity
belts and more.
www.stockroom.com

Temptations
Tantalizing sex toy
supplier which sells a
large BDSM selection,
such as spreader bars,
rope and restraints, fetish
furniture, cock and ball
toys, medical sex toys and
much more
www.temptationsdirect.
co.uk

Tabooboo
Fun site selling costumes,
spankers, restraints and
bondage tape
www.tabooboo.com

UberKinky
Extreme sex toys, BDSM
and bondage gear,
fetishwear, and medical
and electro sex aids.
www.uberkinky.co.uk

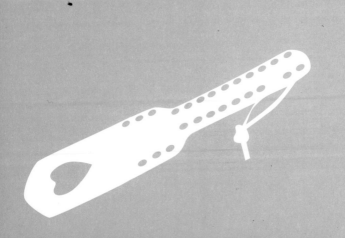